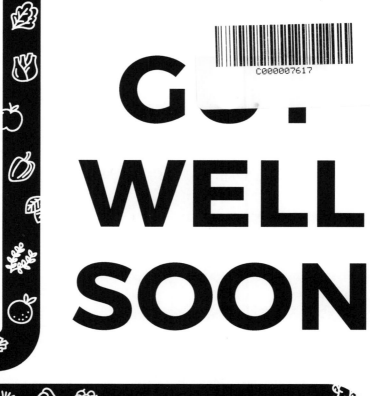

GUT WELL SOON

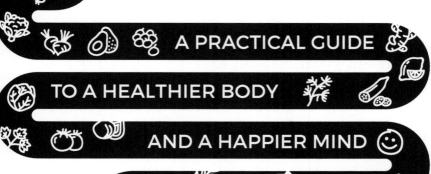

A PRACTICAL GUIDE

TO A HEALTHIER BODY

AND A HAPPIER MIND ☺

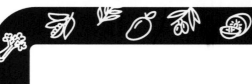

CATHERINE
ROGERS

Gut Well Soon

First published in 2019 by

Panoma Press Ltd
48 St Vincent Drive, St Albans, Herts, AL1 5SJ, UK
info@panomapress.com
www.panomapress.com

Book layout by Neil Coe.

Printed on acid-free paper from managed forests.

ISBN 978-1-784521-56-1

A CIP catalogue record for this book is available from the British Library.

This book is available online and in bookstores.

Dedication

For Mia, my youngest daughter who, at age 12, asked me to write down everything I know as blogs then encouraged me each week until I did.

Who knew it would end up as this book!

Testimonials

As we uncover the hidden world of the microbiome one thing is becoming clear: it is a bridge between our health, and the health of our environment. We now know that our diet and lifestyle including exercise, stress resilience, sleep and exposure to pollution impact the health of our gut bacteria, and this book explores how, and offers practical solutions for regaining your health.

Benjamin I. Brown, ND, author, *The Digestive Health Solution*

I loved – loved – the book overall. So interesting, so timely and so informative.

Suzanne Brais, interested and informed Mum

So, I think I learned about the importance of gut health. Certainly, I learned a lot about how the foods that I eat affect my gut health and therefore affect my performance and my wellbeing. I found that my understanding of what was happening during the Reset Your Gut course was really supported by reading Gut Well Soon *and all the research I could read about in that book, and actually just understanding the processes at work through the different weeks. So yes, I think I did learn a lot but particularly about my own body and what it really thrives off, what doesn't suit it so well and what helps me to be in the best possible health.*

Anon

Gut Well Soon is a little gem! A simple, practical, supremely helpful reference book packed full of excellent advice, tools and tips for you to reset your health and elevate your wellbeing. It is very straightforward and easy to read and digest (no, not a pun!), a handy reference guide you can pick up and read at any time. Absolutely crammed with superb advice, support and help and takes a fresh approach to health and wellness which is aligned to the school of 'Integrative Medicine'. Love this! Leading the way in promoting good gut health in the UK!

Belinda Furneaux-Harris, founder, Branded & Unstoppable.

A great book for anyone wishing to get their health back on track by addressing the cause of many health problems – the gut.

Rose Humphries, satisfied customer

Gut Well Soon looks at topics from all angles and backs up opinions with reference to scientific research, relating to both conventional and functional medicine. It isn't preachy, just common sense when faced with the facts. This is the real strength of the book – and I don't think the targets/suggestions are daunting, the tone of the book is relaxed, friendly and supportive. An inspirational and practical guide to a happy gut and happy mind!

C Jones, Pilates instructor

Loved it. A comprehensive and excellent summary of how to live a happy and healthier life, whatever your starting point. Well referenced, clearly and simply written… covering many complicated and controversial issues… with a focus on nutrition and the importance of the gut. Dispelling many myths and sticking to facts. A page-turner for anyone interested in health and wellness/wanting to live their life to its full potential/increasing their quality of life/ wanting more energy... the list goes on. An addictive read for anyone who wants to better understand the 'why behind the what' of cutting edge (or current/latest) health opinion and advice. I do much of this already but definitely plan to attempt RYG, especially to remove dairy and alcohol for a 4-week trial and see if we feel better/have more energy. Son has been on antibiotics and husband has an autoimmune disorder, daughter loves meat and not fish, so fascinating for them too.

**Clare Cocoran, mum of three, biochemistry BSc
with an interest in health and nutrition**

I enjoyed reading the book, I learned some new things about how my diet and lifestyle choices have a direct impact on both my mental and physical health and how crucial gut health is for overall health. I particularly enjoyed the last chapter due to the positive tone, it gives the reader hope that they can actively make changes to their lifestyle to decrease risks for various diseases.

Deanne, student, London

Topically addresses the public curiosity on the emerging field of the gut microbiome and reinforces the perspective of the functional approach to medicine. We can all do a little less with drugs, and a little more attention to our health. The summary points at the end of the chapters are also helpful to recap on the key concepts.

Amy Kao, studying for a DPhil (PhD) on microbiome and schizophrenia

I thought the book was super interesting and thought provoking. It doesn't seek to impose a view but rather give a balanced and understandable point of view. It simplifies what others seek to make very complicated. This book really got me thinking, clearing much of the deliberate fog that exists about taking personal control of your wellness.

Charles Bevan, 57-year-old company director

The summing up at the end of each chapter and the occasional anecdotes that are thrown in… are absolutely amazing.

Raymond Ho, experimental psychology student

I thought the book was friendly and informative, not at all preachy which can be how some health books can come across. Everything was clear and well explained. I think the repetition of points, eg sleeping well, exercising and drinking water came up in a lot of sections, which was great because each section could be read alone to recap what you need to be doing without having to read the whole book over again! I really liked the bit on exercise (Chapter 3) and found the bit on exam results, concentration and memory so interesting. I also like how the book is honest about where studies are inconclusive.

Juliette Perry, athlete

I do definitely consider my activity and nutrition, but there are lots of little tips in Gut Well Soon that I am going to try to take on board... eating more organic, considering the 'dirty dozen' food list, trying again to really reduce my sugar intake (this is the one big area I really fall down on) and sleep... I just don't get enough of it.

Teresa Devitt, physiotherapist

This is a highly readable and informative book which has answered many of the questions I had about gut health and how it affects my body and mind. I feel confident to put the ideas into action and will certainly look at the Reset Your Gut programme. It feels like the author really knows her stuff and has fully researched the latest scientific and medical research and made it accessible to the everyday reader. I would highly recommend this book to anyone wanting to take their physical and mental health into their own hands to create positive change in their life.

Linda Hamill, nurse

Gut Well Soon is engaging, accessible and beautifully illustrates how easy it can be to take your health into your own hands!

Caitlin, biomedical science undergraduate

This book empowered and encouraged me to make lifestyle changes which have boosted my mental and physical health.

Jane Pares Edney, Ocean Spirit

It's excellent and very timely. This topic is of interest to everyone, that is the power of the book. You don't have to be 'unwell' to buy this book and benefit from it. It's a book that will influence your lifestyle choices in subtle ways every day. It's a must read for anyone who is interested in living a fulfilled and informed life.

Connie Brown, professional coach and learning and development specialist

Acknowledgements

My personal gratitude and debt to all my teachers along the way who have helped develop my knowledge base and encouraged me to be more curious. Martyn Wyse, John Grinder, Dr Sarah Rakovshik and her team at Oxford University: Tamara and Peter Donn, Dr Sarah McKay and Dr Sarah Leung.

Jenny Philips, who has shown me what an inspired well-trained biochemist and cancer survivor can do when they become a nutritionist. Dr Grant, who is living true to the functional and integrative medic path. Anthony Hayes, whose depth of knowledge about vitamins and minerals is amazing, and Dr Jerome Poupel for consistently thinking outside the box and inspiring me to do the same; they both use muscle testing for backing up their diagnosis, an amazing skill. Sophie Lamb, who has helped nurse my migraines with her herbal tinctures. Dr Tanya Malpass, another cancer survivor who has allowed me to quote her blog and through her dedication to eating well has been an inspiration. Dr Isabelle Jacobsen and Ben Brown for their insightful and wise comments and Avani Hurribunce for sharing her experience of reversing diabetes. Charlotte Simpkins, Dan Williams, Jake Peek, Simon Trimmer, Emma Hillan, Laura Cutter, Jack Joseph and Juliette Perry for keeping the accompanying online course *Reset Your Gut* on track while I drafted and redrafted!

Lucy Benyon, who in the early stages helped propel my blogs into the embryo of chapters and Mindy Gibbins-Klein for being my book's midwife, easing it into the world. This project, the book and the online course would not have been possible without the highly motivated, intelligent, challenging and curious interns from Oxford University. Words fail me… as they often did when they consistently exceeded the barriers on delivery. Special thanks go to Matei Marin for early mind nodes and insightful edits and Man Him Ho for his marketing input and our discussions on Cochrane systematic reviews. Caitlin Ashcroft and Dr Amy Kao for unshakeable enthusiasm and positivity, in particular

I would like to thank Caitlin for inspiring the book title, she has an undeniable talent with words! Sophie Hubbard, Deanne Clarke, Sichen Liu for their amazing work ethic, curiosity and humour. What a team!

My clients, who are a constant inspiration to me: first, they bravely take the step to obtain help, and second, they work hard at changing how they think, behave and feel, get more sleep, eat better and attempt to be less stressed – no small achievement, but always rewarding. A special mention to all the ladies at the High Wycombe Family Support group from whom I have learned so much, and Debbie Dust who does an amazing job steering the group, spurred on by her inspiring Christian faith.

Friends who have cajoled and encouraged me along the way. Regina Mabon for her unending curiosity and fun, laughing with me over being a 'flexitarian'. Belinda Furneaux-Harris, Courtney Brennan, Anna Usher, Sally Chilvers and Amanda Carr for their constant encouragement and belief.

All those who have read a draft and given me their honest feedback or just listened to my ideas and given me some of their own. Teresa Devitt, my talented physio, and Irene Smith and Emily Fletcher who both have a great line in supportive listening. Annabel Nicoll who has been on the gut journey from the beginning, Georgina Mullins for her practical feedback, Nicola McLintock, Fergus Murison and Laura Farey for improving the Exercise chapter, Claudia Jones and Clare Cocoran for constructive feedback that moved the book along. Naomi Morten for words of wisdom born from 40 years as a midwife. Jane Pares Edney for an amazing early editing job (loved her comments) and early morning yoga. Kate Parsons for her inspirational drawing. Mike Annesley for his consistently patient technical support. Hamish Leng for the gluten banter. David Carr for removing exclamation marks! Alice Carr for helping early on in the RYG journey and Wendy Rowland Payne, Diahaan Gibbs, Rosanne Murison and Alison Asby for 11th hour advice on the book title and the reality of marketing!

To all my gorgeous, tolerant friends and family who have thought I am off on some hare-brained scheme again… well I was! I apologise for my preoccupation and hope that if you read it you will understand how all-consuming it has been!

Dr Helen MacMullen for being inspirational in the way she chooses to live her life and helped me to stand up and write what I believe in. Dr Isabelle Jacobson, Sam Palmer Endean, Nick Warner, Victoria Day, Jessica Tennant, Suzanne Brais, Mary Ann Stewart, Camilla Leask, Bex Potter, Tim Anderson, Amy Fennell, Mike Annesley, Connie Brown, Kate Peel, Linsey Potter, Pip Wels, Julia Farey, Vicky Clokey, Julia Kirkham, Kathy Smallwood, Kate Borthwick, Lucia Simon, Harriet Hancock, Emma Cripwell and Michelle Wathes. I thank you all for your support.

My husband Chris, who has patiently watched me tap away and quietly suggested I should eat and sleep. He is my rock and my backbone, without him I could not have come this far. Finally, my children Jack, Annie and Mia who are the lights in my life and without whom I would not be complete. Thank you for bearing with Mum while she researched and embarrassed you with her enthusiasm. Our kitchen is a different place from three years ago, and whilst there has been resistance along the way, I could not have come this far without your loving support and gentle humour.

Thank you from the bottom of my heart.

Contents

This book has been fully researched and all the references are easily available from www.ryghealth.com and www.maphealthsolutions.com

Introduction

In the chaos of 21st century life, looking after your health can easily fall to the bottom of a long, long list of priorities. Between the pressures of work, home-life, personal goals and the expectations of our nearest and dearest, trying to change your habits and improve your lifestyle may seem like a mountain that simply isn't worth scaling.

Why bother?

With our current understanding of the human body, not to mention recent advances in medical technology, reaching never before seen heights, what's the point in slaving away at the gym or grappling with 'health foods' you probably can't even pronounce when seemingly the solution to all your health problems is just a doctor's appointment away? We've created a culture in which our physical (and indeed mental) wellbeing only becomes important when something starts going seriously wrong.

While we all *know* our lifestyle choices – diet, sleeping habits, activity levels and environmental factors – affect our health, we don't necessarily consider the impact of our daily habits until they're seen through the lens of a formal, and often scary, medical diagnosis. Unfortunately, with chronic illnesses such as coronary heart disease, diabetes, mental health disorders and age-related conditions such as Alzheimer's on the rise, it's becoming increasingly clear that this 'reactive' approach to health is simply not working. As one world-weary British NHS consultant said to me: "[Doctors] are here to put out fires when, really, we should be building a culture in which those fires never get lit in the first place."

Are you willing to act before you get an illness? Do you want to live life to the full? Are you fed up with all the 'health noise' and want simplicity, or do you have an underlying condition that you want to help? Or maybe you are an athlete looking for peak performance or have low energy or are depressed? If any of these questions resonate with you, this book is for you. Even if you are a sceptic, this book is full of references so you can check out the facts and kindly provide feedback!

So what can we do?

In recent years, a growing proportion of the medical community has been moving towards 'functional medicine': a systems-based approach to healthcare that focuses on identifying and addressing the *causes* of disease rather than simply treating the symptoms. The Institute for Functional Medicine sets the gold standard globally for education, training and clinical practice for practitioners in functional medicine. They are addressing directly the growing cost and exponential growth of chronic disease and are showing with research and inspiring clinical practice that functional medicine can reverse this trend. Dr Dan Lukaczer at the conference Applying Functional Medicine in Clinical Practice said it is essential to look at why body systems are not working well and not just treat symptoms, and Dr Joel Evans emphasised it is by changing conditions (diet, environment, sleep, stress) that enables chronic disease to change and improve.

Conventional medicine has strived to ensure they 'do no harm' but through circumstances, like lack of time and funding, they typically focus on 'quick-fix' (often drug-based) solutions to health problems, often without considering the underlying factors responsible for those issues. Doctors are trained to give a name to a symptom[1] and treat accordingly; the interaction of the whole human body is not their territory. There is a disconnect between what doctors are taught and what we know will help reverse chronic disease: good nutrition, sleep, stress reduction and exercise, and as discussed at length by doctors at the conference for functional medical practitioners, sometimes even they don't realise what they don't know. An exact and precise knowledge is useless sometimes if we are treating symptoms in isolation and not looking at both mental and physical health at the same time.

Physicians and scientists are brilliant and are trained for example to focus on a specific neurotransmitter, but isolated knowledge is useless unless we focus on the whole ecosystem of our bodies. Doctors do have the answers in some situations where we need an operation or a pill to decrease unpleasant symptoms, but encouragingly functional medicine practitioners (including doctors, nutritionists, physiotherapists etc) are coming to realise that a patient's lifestyle can act as both a cause *and* a potential solution to many physical and mental ailments and that pills do not always need to become a way of life.

Our modern lifestyles may be killing us, but it could be the secret to saving us too. The aim of functional medicine is to educate people about the importance of, and ways of implementing, habits and lifestyle practices to keep you fit and healthy, and prevent chronic conditions, both now and in decades to come.

So how do I qualify to write this book? Three reasons: personal experience of looking for a solution to a long-term health problem; working in the mental health field; and my inherent curiosity about the latest 'health' claims.

So firstly, over the past 40 years I have suffered badly from migraines and in-between the pain I have sought out every solution from both mainstream and less mainstream providers. So, what worked? You guessed it… a functional medicine approach, and you will hear other stories in this book where conditions are relieved and sometimes completely disappear by taking the same approach. After years of being told I would have to take strong drugs for the rest of my life (migraines are the third most common disease in the world affecting one in seven people[2]) three or four times a week, I started looking at what my body was not absorbing and the underlying causes of my migraines. In brief (as the whole migraine journey is another book), I managed through functional tests (Chapter 11) to find out in what ways my body was deficient and out of balance and changed my lifestyle accordingly.

Secondly, I work with people with mental health challenges. I have been lucky enough to be trained in a mainstream way in CBT at Oxford University, but through other modalities and clinical work I have realised that whenever a patient engaged in their physical health as well as talking therapies and/or drugs, their recovery was quicker and longer lasting. Of course, my observations were purely anecdotal, so I decided to investigate why. Whilst we know at some level that mental health is affected by what we eat, how much exercise we do, and our stress levels, I wanted to investigate the science. The evidence is all in this book; there is an undeniable connection between physical and mental health especially the microbiome, which is the technical word for the bacteria in your gut (see Chapter 1). It has made me even more passionate about helping those with mental health challenges to move forward.

For this reason, alongside this book I have developed, with the help of dieticians, nutritionists, doctors, scientists, a recipe writer and a team of enthusiastic interns from Oxford University, the online *Reset Your Gut* programme (www.ryghealth.com). I will mention the course in this book as something for you to consider and I make no apology for this; gut bacteria and its role in human health is an explosive area of modern scientific research and it is becoming increasingly obvious that gut health plays a vastly underappreciated role in physical and mental wellbeing. Just see how much research has been done on the microbiome (gut bacteria) since 2015!

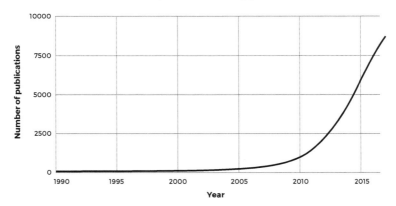

Microbiome publications by year since 1990

The RYG programme is not just a selection of recipes, it is a carefully put together healthy eating plan that is designed to rebalance your microbiome and give your body all the things that it needs, especially your gut bacteria (full details in Chapter 1).

So, with this wealth of information at our fingertips it's often difficult to work out what positive changes look like. Wherever you turn there seems to be a new diet plan or supplement promising to make you 'happier and healthier' and the internet is full of 'uncontrolled' information. At the opposite end of the spectrum you have the dense, jargon-filled (and often difficult to find) academic papers that throw you in at the deep end with statistics, methods and results, leaving you with an aching brain and no greater understanding of whatever it was you wanted to read about in the first place.

So thirdly, this is where I come in.

This book is my attempt to navigate the turbulent waters of health and wellness and explore the science underpinning the health claims and misconceptions we've all heard before but never really understood.

For me, I started with articles published in the popular media (eg *Huffington Post, Daily Mirror, Daily Mail, Independent* etc) and then looked at original research papers and conferences where experts in a particular field present their findings. I was shocked to discover how frequently the original scientific studies were distorted by the press. Of course, this is understandable – the constant news cycle creates a demand to pull traffic to your paper or website or product and what better way to do that than with attention-grabbing, pseudoscientific headlines? Sadly it is a fact that even solid research conclusions take time to filter through to the busy medical profession. In this book I hopefully speed this process up by bringing the information directly to you.

True science is always pushing back the frontiers of what we know and understands that new evidence may emerge that could change the current thinking. Remember when we thought the world was flat? That Aids was contracted by a handshake? That it was OK to drink and drive?

So, in this book I reserve the right for the science and opinion I have stated to be modified in the future, and I welcome any developments in our understanding of what could help us achieve healthier bodies and happier minds. I have included smaller studies for consideration as it is sometimes small insights that can start big changes.

I am clearly not in the camp that says if science can't find out how something works, it cannot be true… however I would encourage you to set your BS meter high when reading the latest 'health news'. Whilst popular diets and some medical terminology can become buzz words and misrepresent the facts, I also see that correct information, well presented, can be the engine for positive change. This book explains the reasons why healthy eating, sleep, avoiding stress, exercise and being sociable are the way to a healthier body and a happier mind.

I hope I have struck a good balance between presenting scientific data and peer reviewed journals that people do not normally read and anecdotes that science does not yet accept!

For example I will be looking at:

- Why should I be eating 5+ servings of fruit and vegetables per day?

- Do I really need to avoid fat, sugar and everything else that I love?

- Why do we sleep and how much should I be getting?

- What is the best way of dealing with mental health problems?

- Are antioxidants what they are purported to be by their marketeers and the media?

- Does taking omega-3 really promote intelligence?

- What is my microbiome, and why should I reset it?

I'll be exploring all of these (and many more) to arm you with the tools you need to make proactive, informed and effective changes to your current lifestyle. From the importance of good nutrition and gut health in mind-body wellbeing, to exercise, stress and how to look after an aging brain, I'll be taking you on a journey through the fact and fiction (and several grey areas!) of the wellness world and looking at the 'why' behind the 'what' of current health advice.

Hopefully, if I've done my job well, you'll begin to see just how much you stand to gain from taking control of your health and tackling problems *before* they arise rather than relying on a doctor's prescription to keep you going. I have written the book with integrity, and I am not being paid to publish any of this material, so the only possible bias is my own!

The references in the book are available listed by chapter on my websites: **www.ryghealth.com** and **www.maphealthsolutions.com**. This will help you find them as you can copy and paste!

Knowledge is power, and I wholeheartedly believe that we all have the power to have a huge impact on our health simply by learning to listen to our bodies and adapt our habits accordingly. Modern life has shifted away from the middle, and we need to re-centre our lifestyles. We are in the midst of a major medical paradigm shift and one that, in my view, could revolutionise what it means to live a healthy, balanced and fulfilled life.

CHAPTER 1

Why your gut bacteria is so important

In the introduction I mentioned briefly the importance of a healthy gut, and we will now be looking in more detail at why having diverse and balanced gut bacteria is so important for your health. Hopefully this is not new to you (but it's all right if it is!) as gut health really is an emerging area of research and healthcare. Indeed, it's something that medical practitioners are becoming quite evangelical about; poor gut health is now being linked to so many health problems. Human cells only make up 43% of your body's cell count, the rest are microscopic colonies and they are essential to your health[1]. Believe it or not, you are more microbe than human. Professor Sarkis Mazmanian, a microbiologist, says: "What makes us human is our own DNA, plus the DNA of our gut microbe" – disrupt them and you will know about it!

What is the microbiome?

Recently, there has been a sea change in the field of human biology. Functional medicine practitioners are beginning to see people more like ecosystems, rather like rainforests and coral reefs, made up of many different organisms. There is a growing recognition that you are not just a mammal, you are an organism which is made up of trillions of different microbes (invisible bacteria, viruses and fungi). The term 'microbiome' is used to refer to the community of microbes you have living on and in your body and I will also call it 'gut bacteria' in this book.

You may be aware that your skin hosts microbes but your gut hosts most of your microbes, and they provide you with a range of beneficial effects. Microbes help you to digest food, with some estimates that bacteria provide up to 15% of your required calories by breaking down food that you cannot do yourself[3]. Certain microbes produce important signalling molecules[3], while others can help with your immune cell development[4]. Given all these amazing functions, it's not surprising that Dr Eamonn Quigley, former president of the American College of Gastroenterology, referred to the gut microbiome as 'the forgotten organ'!

Diversity is key

When it comes to your gut bacteria, diversity is everything: various studies have found that a broader range of bacteria in the gut is better for human health[3]. Obese people[5] and those people who suffer from asthma[6] and allergies are more likely to have less diverse gut bacteria and may find that they are tired, lethargic and lacking in energy[7]. This could of course contribute to mental health challenges when you find you do not have the energy needed for a fulfilling and happy existence, and there is growing evidence (see Psychobiotics section below) that encouraging a healthy microbiome has a positive effect on your mental health.

Functional medical practitioners are realising that anything that reduces the diversity of the gut bacteria, like antibiotics[8] and excessively high levels of hygiene[9], are the precursors to many inflammatory conditions (Chapter 6) and need to be tackled with lifestyle changes. They realise the significance of the trillions of organisms that live inside have on your mental and physical health. The microbiome can exert an indirect influence on the expression of your genes by producing small molecules such as short chain fatty acids (eg acetate) that interact with your DNA. We are losing bacteria that have been used for centuries to switch your genes on and off (this area of study is called epigenetics) and to express your genetic code.

A major contributor to the decrease in bacteria is our western diet: we eat less and less fibre and this is the fuel for your gut bacteria[10]. Scientists are already looking at setting up a 'bacteria bank' to preserve specific microbial strains that our modern lifestyle is making extinct so that we can repopulate our guts with good organisms in the future!

The good bacteria survive by feeding from the fibre we eat, and they are essential to crowd out bacteria that cause infection and create metabolic products that allow you to thrive. For example, they produce B vitamins which send signals to your body via other molecules in an intricate biological process to produce short chain fatty acids, which in turn reduces inflammation and helps the lining of the gut to stay intact. They also activate the production of neurotransmitters that help determine amongst other things our mood – so essential for a happier mind!

It is estimated 70% of the body's immune system is located in your gut, ie the gut-associated lymphoid tissue (GALT)[11]. This system is supported by your gut microbiome. You may have heard the terms 'good bacteria' and 'bad bacteria'. These terms are misleading as it is the proportion, rather than just the type, of each bacteria that is crucial in the biome. There are, indeed, 'bad' bacteria – such as *Salmonella* – that cause disease.

However, in gut bacteria balance is the key as to whether a bacterial species will grow or reduce enough to cause a problem for us. As we will see in the chapter on drugs, antibiotics can reduce the diversity of the microbiome, thus enabling the population of bad bacteria to expand[12,13].

This could then affect your mental (depression) and physical (IBS) health if not addressed with appropriate nutrition and products that introduce and promote a healthy microbial balance (see my *Reset Your Gut* programme outlined below).

For example, by eating a diet full of sugar and excessive saturated fat, you can alter the balance between bacteria such as Bacteroides (B) and Firmicutes (F) bacteria. F are used by your body to digest fats and B are used to digest fibre; a poor diet will encourage the F bacteria population to increase, thus dictating if your body is lean or obese. Obesity-associated microbes can affect your insulin resistance (a precursor for diabetes), fat deposition, metabolism, appetite, and even cause inflammation. The research so far has been done with mice[14], but I am sure it will not be long until research establishes the link in humans.

Scientists are becoming increasingly interested in the connection between the gut and the brain, and there is now significant evidence that a compromised biome can affect our mental health (depression and anxiety[15]). Dr Sarah McKay, an Oxford-educated neuroscientist and an increasingly influential brain health commentator, who specialises in translating brain science research into simple and actionable strategies for health and wellbeing, suggests that "a healthy balance of gut microbes can contribute to normal behaviour and a well-functioning immune system and a poor balance of microbes disrupts the gut-brain signalling pathways".

Overwhelmingly, the message is that what we eat and how we treat our gut bacteria will influence our health. Over 400 diverse nutritional experts from over 40 countries agreed when they met in New York at the True Health Initiative[16] that eating a Mediterranean-style diet (see Chapter 2) was the way forward. I find it encouraging that these paleo exponents or vegan enthusiasts all agreed that fresh vegetables and fruit are fundamental to your mental and physical health, whatever their area of expertise. I find it interesting that they all agreed on the basics of a good diet, and this highlights the impact the media and vested interests have in distorting this basic consensus and attempting to confuse us!

The RYG programme follows this simple approach.

And if you take their advice, good news! The fibre in the fruit and veg will affect which bacteria dominate in your microbiome and this in turn will influence your immune system. It will support your ability to release the nutrition from your food and give you energy to supply the body's systems with the nutrients they require to function properly. Check out Chapter 11 to see what tests you can do to see if your gut bacteria are out of balance.

We all have compromised microbiomes

Our modern world has left many of us with compromised microbiomes. Our western lifestyle is very different from the hunter-gatherer environments that we evolved in[17]. Not surprisingly, many of us are paying the price with our health. There are a variety of lifestyle factors that have been shown to influence the gut microbiome – let's look at these next.

Food

Eating less processed food, additives and reducing your intake of trans fats (see Chapter 2) and refined sugars will all help to improve the levels of healthy bacteria in your gut. The gut microbiome has been shown to be highly responsive to even short-term alterations in diet[18]. It is understood that foods rich in processed fats and sugars can alter the composition of the gut bacteria resulting in an imbalance that may disrupt bowel movements. To prove this point, Professor Tim Spector, author of *The Diet Myth: The Real Science Behind What We Eat*, challenged his student son Tom to only eat McDonald's for ten days. The result was that Tom lost 1,400 bacterial species from his gut – almost a third of his microbiome[19].

If we want to encourage good bacteria, it is clear that we need a balanced diet that is rich in plant-based foods and dietary fibre[20,21] (more on this later).

Poor sleep

Scientists investigating the impact that the microbiome has on circadian rhythms and quality of sleep have found that there is a link between gut health and your shut-eye[22]. Disruptions to the circadian rhythms, perhaps due to jet lag or insomnia, can cause alterations in the body's microbial ecosystem, and over the long term this can make you far more vulnerable to metabolic imbalances, glucose intolerance and weight gain.

There is also evidence to suggest that the irregular breathing associated with obstructive sleep apnoea (OSA) may affect the quality and balance of bacteria in your body. In one study researchers disrupted the breathing patterns of mice for six weeks and subsequently observed significant changes to the diversity and makeup of their microbiomes[23]. Scientists are investigating whether this is a two-way street... does a compromised gut microbiome cause OSA?

Stress

There is a strong link between the brain and your gut involving hormonal and nerve pathways. This connection forms the basis of your gut-brain axis and this relationship is bidirectional: your gut health (and microbiome composition and diversity) can have a direct impact on your mental and emotional wellbeing, and your mental and emotional state can impact your gut bacteria. For instance, being under constant stress can change the balance and diversity of gut microorganisms, which can have a negative impact on the body's immune system[24].

According to the American Psychological Association (APA), 95% of the body's feel-good hormone serotonin supply is produced by your gut bacteria[25]. Research has found that encouraging growth of your good gut bacteria by consuming prebiotics (see section coming up) could play a role in treating depression and anxiety[26]. The growing recognition of the interplay between the gut bacteria and our mental health promises novel and exciting developments regarding treatment options for common maladies including stress, depression and anxiety. This is why I always encourage my clients with mental health challenges to not only seek help via talking therapies and perhaps appropriate drugs, but to also consider the RYG programme for a healthier body and a happier mind.

Inflammation

Your stomach and its microbiome are particularly vulnerable to stress, and you may well have experienced stress as tummy cramps or butterflies before a date or an interview. When your brain registers stress, it releases a peptide hormone called corticotropin releasing factors (CRF) which can result in inflammation in your gut; chronic stress has therefore been linked to anxiety and depression[27].

Inflammation (see Chapter 6), sometimes known as the 'silent killer', is the catalyst for many chronic illnesses. Research published in the journal of *Nutritional Clinical Practice* revealed that when your gut bacteria is affected by inflammation, it affects your metabolism, immune system and energy levels[28] (see Chapter 10).

Gut permeability

Inside your bowel there is a single layer of cells known as the epithelium that acts as a barrier between the contents of your gut and the rest of your body. The epithelial layer prevents harmful bacteria and substances passing from the bowel into your bloodstream. When this barrier becomes compromised, and your microbiome balance is disrupted, these toxins are free to circulate in your body, causing you all sorts of health problems.

Commonly, this has become known as leaky gut syndrome (LGS), though it is referred to as gut hyperpermeability in the medical community. Being under stress can contribute towards gut permeability, as can the consumption of some fatty foods [29,30] (see Chapter 6 for full details).

Antibiotics

Antibiotics are very effective in blasting any harmful pathogenic/disease-causing bacteria, but unfortunately they destroy good bacteria too (see Chapter 7). Studies carried out both in the UK and Sweden have revealed that healthy patients who take a week-long course of antibiotics are at risk of compromising their gut microbiome for up to a year. Volunteers who took certain kinds of antibiotics not only displayed a significant drop[3] in their levels of butyrate (a great fatty acid that lowers oxidative stress and inflammation in the intestines[31]) but also a sustained effect, with the diversity of their microbiome taking some months to return to its previously balanced state.

This isn't to say that you shouldn't take a course of antibiotics under the advice of your GP to treat a bacterial infection, but you might just want to think about supporting your system through such times by taking the correct probiotic and consuming lots of prebiotic foods that will promote the growth of your good bacteria (see supplements suggested in the *Reset Your Gut* programme via www.ryghealth.com and definition of pre- and probiotics later in this chapter).

Smoking and air pollution

Smoking and toxic chemicals in the air you breathe can cause alterations in your gut microbiome composition. The chemicals inhaled in cigarette smoke and other air-borne pollutants are trapped in mucus in your lungs, which are then brought up from your lungs by the rhythmic motion of cilia – minute hair-like formations which line our airways. This mucus is then swallowed and enters the digestive system, where the chemicals it contains interact with the microbes of your gut. Evidence suggests that alterations in bacterial composition caused by air pollution, and particularly smoking[32] may increase the risk of developing Crohn's Disease (CD) and Inflammatory Bowel Disease (IBD)[20,33].

Early years

A correlation has been identified between birth by C-section and the development of conditions such as asthma and diabetes and even obesity[34,35]. This may be due to the fact that babies born this way are not exposed to their mother's microbiome during natural vaginal delivery. Anecdotally it would appear the science is being interpreted in different ways on the 'rock face' of maternity wards. Upon investigation I found one local health authority gave instructions for babies to be swabbed with the mother's vaginal fluid after a caesarean birth, and another said that there is not enough evidence and advises against this practice.

This area of research on the connection between a compromised microbiome and caesarean birth is in its infancy and you may wish to watch the film on the website www.microbirth.com to gain more information.

After birth – either natural or by C-section – bacteria continue to colonise an infant's intestine, helping the immune system to recognise bacterial allies and enemies. Research from the University of California found that close to 30% of the beneficial bacteria in a baby's intestinal tract come directly from the mother's breast milk in breast-fed babies[36].

In her book *Healthy Food, Healthy Gut, Happy Child*, Dr Maya Shetreat-Klein claims that sanitising our children's lives with cleaning products, pesticides and medication is preventing them from developing a healthy and balanced microbiome. She says we should be encouraging our kids to spend time outside in green open spaces to build up their healthy bacteria[37].

Age matters

Scientists have found that the composition of your gut microbiome changes as you age and the bacteria in your guts may play a role in determining our immunity, cognitive function and muscle mass retention[38,39] over time. The composition of gut bacteria in the elderly has also been shown to be sensitive to diet, community integration, and mental and physical decline (ie whether a person lives in a community or in a care home)[39].

How to reset your microbiome

Research comparing the microbiota of populations in Africa with European ones has demonstrated that the western diet has caused a reduction in our microbial variety as well as the loss of bacteria potentially involved in conferring protection against certain diseases[40]. While those living in rural African communities might have tens of thousands of varieties of microbes in their gut, in the west we have a lot less[41]. We know that overcleanliness, a poor diet, medication, pollution and stress are all having a negative impact on our microbiome. The good news is that we can test (see Chapter 11 Functional Tests) to see the state of our microbiome and there are simple lifestyle modifications we can make to reverse this trend and create better gut health. By healing our gut and rebalancing our microbiome this can help your body and brain function at an optimal level.

Reset your gut

In the UK abdominal and pelvic pain account for more hospital admissions than any other health emergency. Before you become a statistic check out the *Reset Your Gut* programme at www.ryghealth.com.

This, as mentioned in the introduction, is an online course created to help you establish and promote a balanced gut microbiome by following a structured and easy-to-follow four-week programme. Approved by nutritionists and used by medical doctors and other health professionals to encourage their patients to reset the balance of their gut bacteria, it is simple and economic and something you could easily incorporate into your busy life.

RYG provides clients with a personalised three meal a day plan and shopping list, and step by step recipes designed to meet all your nutritional needs, and incorporates key foods known to encourage good gut health. Fibre-rich, nutrient-rich and filled with pre- and probiotics your gut will love!

RYG has enabled people to make lasting lifestyle changes rather than following temporary diet regimes or taking expensive products, and you can take your health into your own hands and restore the balance of your microbiome.

In simple terms it works like this: you remove all processed food and inflammatory foods from your diet (see Chapter 2 and Chapter 6) and at the same time introduce anti-inflammatory foods, rich in pre- and probiotics, and glutamine-rich foods that promote gut repair. The RYG programme is based on the Institute of Functional Medicine's 5R Framework for Gut Restoration (for more details see www.ryghealth.com). Working with PhD researchers who are looking at the microbiome in the context of the immune system, schizophrenia, and other areas, I have discovered that our microbiome is definitely not linear. It will respond to good nutritional input at any time and the RYG programme reflects this reality. This approach gives your body back its innate capability to balance your whole system for a healthier body and a happier mind.

Remove inflammatory foods

If you want to restore the diversity of your microbiome and repair damage to the gut wall, it is crucial to eat the right food. If you fancy going the whole hog with a total gut reset, then for a period of time you need to eliminate dairy, gluten, alcohol, sugar (including the fructose found in fruit drinks), caffeine, chlorinated water and processed food. If that sounds too restrictive (after all, you want to have a life still!) just try to reduce these foods and replace them with prebiotics (see below) and plant-based foods. Excessive meat consumption has been linked with colo-rectal cancer[42] and one of the proven ways to improve digestive functioning and microbiome health is by eating more dietary fibre and consuming a predominantly plant-based diet.

Various products have been launched that claim to help you improve the balance of your microbiome. However, Dr Kirstie McLoughlin, who has a PhD looking at how 'adaptive immune system modulates the gut microbiota', says it is important to remember that for some people "the resetting of the microbiome is going to take a consistent lifestyle change", not three or four weeks of taking a product. The science around the microbiome is in its infancy, it may be the most exciting breakthrough for modern medicine, but we still know so little.

You could choose to do a stool test (see Chapter 11). This would identify what the normal bacterial population is in your gut and if you have any inflammatory markers, parasitic pathogens, immune triggers, parasites, or yeasts. You could then get advice from a functional medical practitioner to consider if any of these could be causing you a mental or physical health issue. However, in my opinion the first step before taking any product or doing a stool test would be to follow the *Reset Your Gut* programme which is a practical approach to maintaining a healthy gut via what you are eating.

Fasting

As far as health regimes go, fasting is uncomplicated as it simply involves going without food for between 12 and 30 hours. But did you know that regular fasting could protect your body from harmful bacteria? A study on fruit flies revealed that a genetic 'switch' activated by fasting helped to halt the spread of intestinal bacteria into the bloodstream[43]. Of course, we are not insects, but I have one client who swears that she lifted herself out of depression by not eating 12 hours out of 24 …! See Chapter 13 for more details of the impact fasting can have on your health.

Probiotics

Probiotics are essentially any foods that contain live bacteria that can survive the acid environment of the stomach and then increase the number of good bacteria in the gut. They are incredibly useful to our body, producing vital vitamins that our bodies need and chemicals that can kill diarrhoea viruses. Our gut bacteria, as we are seeing, can, amongst other things, reduce inflammation, the risk of diabetes and heart disease, so it is really important to know which probiotics help the gut bacteria to thrive.

There has been some debate about the effectiveness of pre-prepared manufactured probiotic supplements and some foods sold as probiotics. A study broadcast on the BBC2 programme *Trust Me, I'm A Doctor* revealed that a sample group of people who took probiotic supplements every day for four weeks saw a significant change in one type of healthy gut microbe, whilst volunteers who drank kefir, a fermented drink, saw a rise in a whole family of bacteria which are believed to reduce the symptoms of lactose intolerance and IBS, and to cut the risk of infection (please note the kefir in the RYG programme is made with coconut milk).

Professor Simon Gaisford from UCL school of pharmacy also did an interesting experiment for the BBC series. He tested which commonly available probiotic foods survived the highly acidic environment of the stomach. He wanted to know which foods delivered probiotics to your intestines "so they could support the digestive system, stimulate the immune system and prevent the spread of unhealthy bacteria".

The sauerkraut bacteria did not make it through the stomach; chocolate with probiotic added and kimchee did slightly better, but the only foods that survived the equivalent of being in the stomach for 30 minutes (the same time as a meal takes to digest) were kefir and natural yogurt. Professor Gaisford stated that the fat content of the latter protected them from the acid in the stomach.

Conversely, a study at the William and Mary University in Virginia revealed that students who ate more fermented food such as live unsweetened yoghurt, pickles and sauerkraut, which are high in natural probiotics, exhibited fewer symptoms of social anxiety and neuroticism[44] even if they had a higher genetic risk for the conditions. So maybe the trick is to eat high-quality fermented food with some fat food and on an empty stomach? Further proof of the power your guts could have over your mind!

Ana Valdes at the University of Nottingham found that "the effect of probiotic depends on bacteria that are already present in the gut" and whilst probiotics probably don't permanently change the microbe composition of the gut, when ingested effectively they do directly affect our health in many positive ways.

Prebiotics

Prebiotic foods help beneficial bacteria to thrive in your gut; they are described in scientific literature as a non-digestible food ingredient that promotes the growth of beneficial bacteria in the intestine[45].

You need these bacteria to thrive as they produce the metabolites that influence so many of your bodily functions. Your body cannot produce these metabolites, only your bacteria can by breaking down the fibre that we consume.

Examples of some easily accessible and delicious prebiotics are garlic, onion, asparagus, leek, Jerusalem or globe artichoke, radishes, banana (preferably not fully ripe) and chicory root.

Prebiotics help your body resist gastric acidity, are fermented by intestinal bacteria and stimulate selectively the growth and activity of intestinal bacteria associated with health and wellbeing[46]. There is also some evidence that dietary fibre from wholefoods protects against cardiovascular disease, obesity, and type 2 diabetes and is essential for optimal digestive health[47]. If this not enough evidence to encourage you to up your fibre, then other health benefits ascribed to consuming prebiotic foods are as follows:

- Reduced prevalence and duration of infectious agents and antibiotic-associated diarrhoea

- Reduced inflammation and symptoms associated with inflammatory bowel disease

- Protective effects against colon cancer

- Enhanced bioavailability and uptake of minerals, including calcium, magnesium, and possibly iron

- Promotion of satiety and weight loss and prevention of obesity[47]

New and exciting for my work: psychobiotics

The term 'psychobiotics' is a newly suggested concept to include any compound whose effect on the brain is bacterially mediated[48]. These compounds can include both probiotics, which are live cultures of specific bacteria, as well as prebiotics, which are indigestible fibres that enhance the growth of beneficial gut bacteria. By beneficially manipulating the gut, empirical evidence has shown them to exert anxiolytic (anti-anxiety) and antidepressant effects in various parameters such as emotional, cognitive, systemic and neural indices. This approach has been recognised by the NHS to prevent conditions such as antibiotic-associated diarrhoea (AAD), helping with IBS symptoms and lactose intolerance, as well as other minor gastrointestinal ailments[49].

Exciting research is also being done on mental health where probiotic and prebiotic interventions have been shown to positively affect mood in healthy volunteers. Similarly, in the ongoing field of cognitive psychology, evidence has been accumulating to suggest probiotic and prebiotic ingestion can improve learning and memory, as well as cognitive flexibility[50]. Although this research has not yet been replicated in humans, the numerous examinations in animal models provide extremely promising results for this fascinating topic.

Put simply, you can supplement yourself with psychobiotics through food.

Summing up

- A balanced, varied microbiome is key to maintaining good physical and mental health

- Eat a healthy, natural diet containing probiotics and prebiotics

- Get a good night's sleep and manage your stress levels

- Only take antibiotics if you really need to

- Get your hands dirty, and spend more time outside

The RYG programme is a simple, efficient programme designed to obtain and maintain optimal gut health: www.ryghealth.com.

Go online to get a free booklet called *Guidelines For Rebalancing Your Gut Bacteria.*

Notes:

....

....

....

....

....

....

....

CHAPTER 2

Eat well?
Why should I?

W hat exactly does eating a healthy diet mean to you? Eating well isn't rocket science but it has been complicated with all the different advice available and this has paralysed consumers. Nutrition is a complicated symphony of chemicals and complex to understand. It is common sense that eating a balanced diet of healthy food can truly improve your mental and physical health. You don't need to understand the individual notes, just play the music! Research shows that disease prevention and recovery from injury and surgery improves when supported by proper nutrition.

The most challenging thing about eating well may be that it involves a change in lifestyle, and only you can do this. You may have to change some of the weekly items in your shopping bag, which could initially be hard culturally to change, but it does not mean you can never eat those favourite foods that have been demonised by the media. If you eat healthily 80% of the time, then go ahead and indulge yourself the other 20%! It is all about balance.

In the previous chapter, we looked at how you can protect the diversity of your microbiome with what you eat, and later we look at the impact what you eat has on your mental health.

When it comes to mental and physical wellbeing, you really are what you eat. If you ingest something toxic, your gut communicates that to your brain via the enteric nervous system (ENS) and pushes your body into overdrive as it attempts to protect itself. The ENS is a network of neurons that aids gastrointestinal function and enables the gut to communicate with the brain via the release of biochemicals. To keep your ENS happy, it's essential that you absorb the correct vitamins, minerals and other nutrients from your food to promote optimal gut function and ultimately a healthier body and a happier mind!

What we eat plays a major role in determining the makeup of our microbiome. This, in turn, may alter the production of metabolites that influence our risk of developing many chronic diseases[1]. Improving your diet is a far easier way of controlling the balance of your microbiome than, say, reducing stress, and will inevitably help your mental health as well (see Chapter 4).

To help you get started, we will be examining the impact certain foods can have on your health.

Sugar and carbohydrate

If you're eating relatively well, managing your stress levels and exercising regularly, indulging in the odd doughnut or can of cola isn't a problem. As with everything, moderation is the key and maintaining a balanced approach to your diet and lifestyle is essential. If you take a minute to honestly reflect on your sugar consumption, you may realise you're still eating more than you ought to. Unfortunately, in modern western culture, it's far too easy to consume more sugar than you're consciously aware of due to its abundance in common packaged and processed foods (even those marketed as healthier options).

A BBC documentary *The Truth About Carbs* showed in a graphic way that these common foods are the equivalent to a shocking number of sugar cubes:

- bagel   11

- chocolate muffin   10

- bowl of white rice   20

- bowl of strawberries   4

- jacket potato   19

This representation is too simplistic. You need to look at the quality of the sugar or carbohydrate you are eating as well as the quantity.

A piece of fruit may have the same 'sugar cube' level as a sugary cereal but they have a completely different effect on the body because of the nutrient levels within the food. We need good-quality carbohydrate for our bodies to function, for example a baked potato may be consumed with unsaturated fat and lots of fibrous vegetables, which would reduce the impact on your sugar levels compared to two chocolate muffins! However, you can see from this that just because something does not taste sweet does not mean it has no sugar in it, and it is crucial to understand that any energy in the form of blood sugar, if we do not burn it off, will be stored as fat.

The RYG programme is an excellent approach for keeping blood glucose levels low, providing good-quality carbohydrates and fibre to establish balance in your gut bacteria, and helping your immune system to function effectively.

Let's take a closer look at what else sugar does to your body.

Immune system

A study at Loma Linda University revealed that children who were given 100g of sugar – the equivalent of a litre bottle of fizzy drink – experienced a 40% decrease in the effectiveness of their white blood cells (the immune cells responsible for destroying bacteria). This drop in immunity could last for up to five hours[2].

Waistline

When it comes to piling on the pounds, all calories are not created equal. A study conducted in Norfolk as part of the European Prospective Investigation into Cancer and Nutrition (EPIC) revealed that people who have very sugary diets are 54% more likely to be obese than those who eat very little sugar[3]. (This of course leaves 46% who have a sugary diet who are not obese, so maybe they are more active and burn the sugar off before it is stored as fat? It is difficult to know from the study.)

Cancer risk

While certain body tissues require glucose to survive (eg the brain and red blood cells), there is still a very clear link between excessive consumption of sugar and cancer.

According to Jenny Phillips, a biochemist, nutritionist, type 4 cancer survivor and author of *Eat 2 Outsmart Cancer:* "...all carbohydrate – whether from chocolate, buns, carrots, apples or toast – is broken down into glucose (sugar) which is transported in your bloodstream and used by your cells to provide energy. Cancer cells *love* sugar. They have many more insulin receptors on the cell surface than non-cancer cells and this helps glucose enter the cell, which helps the cancer cell grow. This fact is used to study and locate tumours using MRIs[4]... so, regulating your sugar intake is essential and a vital step to support your body during treatment and recovery...".

Sugar consumption has also been *indirectly* linked with cancer. For instance, a diet rich in refined sugars has been linked with obesity, while being overweight or obese has been directly linked with an increased risk of developing certain cancers (and an increased death rate for all cancers)[5]. There is also evidence that increased sugar intake may be in some way associated with the incidence of colorectal cancer[6].

Unfortunately, the medical community does not always appreciate the link between sugar and cancer. I was shocked when a close friend suffering from cancer was told by her doctor that the most important thing to do was to 'get the calories in her' and forget about nutrition.

Perhaps this illustrates that nutrition is not currently being given the attention it deserves in today's medical education (current medical degrees only offer ten to 24 hours of nutritional education, if they are lucky). Again and again it has been shown that in cases of radical cancer remission patients have often made the same basic dietary changes: eliminating sugar, reducing meat consumption (> 5% of daily intake) and removing refined foods[7].

Advice to 'just fill up on calories', regardless of how empty those calories are, is unbelievable and contrary to the basic premise of medicine that one 'should do no harm'. After all, calorie rich is irrelevant if it is nutrient poor. Many people, not only those with cancer, do not have good nutrition and we are seeing high levels of chronic disease (eg obesity, diabetes, hypertension etc) which studies are showing are linked to dietary and lifestyle choices[8,9].

There are hundreds of thousands of nutritional studies published every year (readily available on PubMed and Google Scholar) that highlight the powerful anti-cancer properties of certain foods. These include, but are not limited to, berries and the cruciferous and allium vegetable family[10]. For example, a study in 2015 investigating why rural Africans display significantly reduced prevalence of common western diseases showed that when this cohort was given an average western diet (rich in meat, dairy, processed food, sugar, salt etc) the amount of inflammatory pro-cancer markers shot up. Conversely, when a group of African-Americans were put on a traditional African diet (beans, peas, lentils, corn, wholegrains etc) their pro-cancer markers displayed a dramatic decrease after just two weeks[11].

Cancer is a natural and common cellular process. Your body contains millions of cells that are continuously replicating and dividing, and it only takes a few mistakes in this copying process – perhaps due to toxins (see Chapter 8 and Chapter 9) or inflammation (see Chapter 6) – for cancerous cells to begin to develop. Most do no harm and are quickly eliminated, provided our immune system is supported by good food, regular exercise and plenty of sleep[12]. However, cancerous cells can become problematic when they start hijacking and feeding from your blood supply, if the composition of your microbiome is severely compromised[13] or if your lifestyle is affecting your body's ability to flush them out.

I often hear people say 'I can't avoid cancer – it's genetic', but according to the UK National Cancer Institute, inherited mutations are thought to play a role in only 5-10% of all cancers, while the remainder can be attributed to a wide number of causes including poor nutrition, stress, and environmental factors. A cancer diagnosis is a terrifying prospect, but you can do something about it – all the more reason to start making positive lifestyle changes now.

Tooth decay

This might seem obvious, but you may want to think twice the next time your children ask for sweets. According to the latest figures from the NHS, around 40,000 youngsters under the age of 18 need to have teeth extracted in hospital every year due to excessive decay. Not only is this traumatic for the children involved, it is also very costly to the health service. Many of these operations could be prevented by reducing sugar intake and improving dental hygiene[14].

Liver damage

Research has shown that regularly drinking sugar-sweetened beverages increases your risk of developing non-alcoholic fatty liver disease, especially if you are overweight[15]. However, as you will see, this does not necessarily mean you're better off sticking to artificially sweetened drinks and food.

Sugar vs artificial sweeteners

Whilst artificial sweeteners were not found to increase the risk of liver disease, research has shown that people who take sweeteners regularly are more vulnerable to glucose intolerance, type 2 diabetes and weight gain[16,17]. A connection has been made, albeit in animal models (primarily mice and fruit flies) between artificial sweeteners and increased appetite through the activation of specific neural pathways linked to hunger. This is thought to occur due to the mismatch between the sweet taste of the artificial sweeteners and its low-calorie content, which sends the body into 'feed me' mode!

Researcher Prof. Greg Neely reported: "When we investigated why animals were eating more even though they had enough calories, we found that chronic consumption of an artificial sweetener actually increases the sweet intensity of real nutritive sugar, and this then increases the animal's overall motivation to eat more food. The pathway we discovered is part of a conserved starvation response that actually makes nutritious food taste better when you are starving"[18].

Subsequent work has shown that artificial sweetener-related glucose intolerance may be caused by alterations in gut flora, and the loss of microbes involved in important sugar metabolism pathways[19] – more on this in Chapter 10.

Sugar and the glycaemic index (GI)

When it comes to watching your sugar intake, it is not just the amount of sugar you are putting into your body that matters but also how fast that sugar then enters your bloodstream.

The glycaemic index (GI) can be used to help you decide which foods you should be incorporating into your diet and which are best to avoid. It is a ranking of carbohydrates on a scale from 0 to 100 that is determined by the extent to which they raise your blood sugar levels after eating. A low GI food (ranking 55 or below) such as yoghurt or beans will deliver sugar into your bloodstream far slower than high GI foods (70 to

100) such as white rice, which will cause a rapid blood sugar spike. The body responds to this by producing insulin, a hormone that functions to lower blood sugar and promote fat storage, cellular replication and growth. Medium GI foods are ranked at 55 to 70.

Certain foods can actually slow the rate of glucose uptake into the bloodstream. For instance, one study revealed that drinking sugar water while eating berries slowed the release of fruit sugar into the blood and prevented the hypoglycaemic dip (the 'sugar crash') compared to drinking sugar water on its own[20]. Confusingly, the same study also found that consuming the sugar water along with natural fruit juice also prevented the exaggerated sugar spike, suggesting there is some component of natural fruit juice that influences the regulation of blood sugar levels (perhaps due to the presence of phytonutrients). However, there was still a sugar spike, and as fruit juice does not contain any fibre it will still increase your blood sugar levels more than whole fruit, so I would recommend sticking to the latter if you want to keep your blood sugar down.

I would encourage you to get a general idea of different levels of GI in different types of foods – a complete database can be found at http://www.diogenes-eu.org/GI-Database/Default.htm or look at www.nhs.uk/common-health-questions/food-and-diet/what-is-the-glycaemic-index-gi/#high-gi-foods.

Please note that foods are only given a GI ranking if they contain carbohydrates. Therefore, most meat, fish, eggs and cheese won't be ranked. Also, the presence of fat and protein in a dish will lower the GI of the GI-rated foods in that dish (eg crisps have a lower GI than baked potatoes as they are prepared using oil).

Fats

Fats are often given a bad name because of their supposed association with weight gain (a view often promoted by the food industry) but eating fat doesn't equal *getting fat*. Indeed, it is far more likely that you will gain weight from eating too many high-GI carbohydrates. It has traditionally been recommended that you get between 20% and 35% of your energy from fats as they have an exceptionally important role to play in your body[21,22]. However, people eating a traditional Mediterranean diet, (largely plant based with monounsaturated fats, see definition below) get more of their daily calories from fat, often up to 45%.

Here is a list of some of the health benefits of fats:

- They help your body to absorb vitamins A, D, E and K

- Fats are instrumental in building cell membranes

- They play a vital role in hormone production

- They are important for the health of your skin, hair and nails[23]

- Fats are also essential for good brain health as the brain is, itself, 60% fat

- They increase satiety, ie they ensure you do not get hungry!

This is why low-fat diets are a *bad idea*. Low-fat products have been promoted by the food industry for a long time on the basis of the connection between the consumption of fats and coronary heart disease. While this link has been identified, perhaps incorrectly (see next section), in the case of *saturated* fats – found in meat, cheese and other animal products – this does not apply to the healthy *unsaturated* fats found in nuts, seeds, olives and avocados.

Unfortunately, the research in this area has been significantly distorted resulting in the general public being told in the past to just 'cut out fat', despite the key role fat plays in supporting optimum body function. It is therefore essential to realise that not all fats are equally beneficial to your health and to learn how to separate the 'good' from the 'bad'.

Let's have a look at the different types of fats.

Saturated fats

Saturated fats are typically solid at room temperature and are found in products such as meats, lard, butter and cheese. It is generally recommended that you limit your daily intake of saturated fats to less than a third of your total fat consumption.

The recommended restriction placed on saturated fat intake is due to the links that have been made between saturated fats, increased cholesterol levels and, ultimately, an increased risk of coronary heart disease. However, this remains an area of fierce debate. Correlation does not always equal causation and no studies have yet definitively indicated that a low saturated fat diet prolongs life (German and Dillard, 2004). In fact, the public health recommendations from the American Heart Association to reduce saturated fat intake to 5-6% of the total calorie intake have been found to have no scientific basis whatsoever, implying we shouldn't necessarily believe everything we're told about saturated fats.

More recent research has suggested that while there is an association between saturated fat and increased cholesterol, it is not the absolute amount of cholesterol in the blood that matters but the balance between 'good' (high density lipoprotein or HDL) and 'bad' (low density lipoprotein, LDL) cholesterol. This ratio is not dependent on the percentage of energy coming specifically from saturated fats, but the relative proportions of dietary fatty acids we're consuming (Khaw et al., 2018). Whilst further research is required to establish exactly which fats are best, advice is to eat saturated fats in moderation.

Where are they found? In meat, dairy and coconut oil. Coconut oil has become very popular and portrayed as a 'superfood' like blueberries and avocado, but it is still a saturated fat and there is little evidence for the 'superfood' health benefits promoted. Like other saturated fats, do include it in your diet, but as Dr St Onge, Associate Professor of Nutritional Medicine at Cornell University, points out, his research that the food industry used to promote the status of coconut oil was based on only one component of coconut oil, the medium chain triglycerides

(MCT) which make up only 13-15% of coconut oil. So please do not believe the marketing hype!

Unsaturated fats

Unsaturated fats are liquid at room temperature and present in vegetable oils, nuts, seeds and fish. These are the 'good guys' of the fat world and it is generally recommended that they make up around two thirds of your daily fat intake and one fifth of our daily energy intake. I would recommend virgin olive oil, as canola, corn, peanut etc may be highly processed.

There are two types of unsaturated fats:

- **Monounsaturated fats**: These fats are fantastic at reducing 'bad' LDL cholesterol and increasing 'good' HDL cholesterol (reference: PubMed: 2649645).

  Where are they found? We can find them in olive oil, sesame oil, avocados and most nuts.

- **Polyunsaturated fats**: Not only do these fats reduce LDL cholesterol but they contain omega-3 and omega-6, essential fatty acids that your body can't produce in sufficient amounts by itself, which are crucial for regulating blood pressure, aiding brain development, boosting the immune system[24] and better cardiovascular health. There is an ongoing discussion about the potential for omega-6 fats to compete with the more beneficial omega-3s, but this is beyond the realm of this book[25].

  Where are they found? In fish such as salmon, trout and mackerel and in sunflower seeds flaxseeds and walnuts.

Trans fats

Trans fats occur naturally in small amounts in some food (eg meat and dairy) but are primarily produced artificially by hydrogenation – a process that uses hydrogen to turn liquid oils into solids. These hardened oils are typically used in products such as margarine and baked goods like crisps.

When consumed in small quantities as part of a balanced diet, trans fats do not pose any major health problems. However, too much can definitely be bad for our health. Trans fats have been proven to raise 'bad' LDL cholesterol, and lower 'good' HDL cholesterol. As noted earlier, high LDL cholesterol level increases the risk of cardiovascular diseases and stroke, while HDL cholesterol level reverses these effects[26], therefore eating too much trans fat can increase our risk of developing coronary heart disease. For this reason, the British government recommends that adults eat less than 5g of trans fats per day[27].

Where are they found? In margarine, and baked goods such as biscuits, cookies and crisps. Regulation changes in the food industry now mean that margarines contain less trans fat than they once did, but if in doubt, check the label for trans fat and/or hydrogenated vegetable oil. Trans fats also occur naturally in some kinds of foods (eg cheese, beef and mutton) at very low levels, but in general I would recommend you try to avoid trans fats when added artificially in foods.

Protein

Proteins are large molecules composed of smaller molecules called amino acids. Proteins are essential to life – they are found in every cell in the body and are used for every cellular process including growth and repair. Some of the 20 or so different types of amino acid can be synthesised within the body from other protein, but some essential amino acids cannot and must therefore be consumed in the food you eat. It is therefore important to consume protein from a variety of sources to ensure that you take in the full range of amino acids. Dietary guidelines suggest you consume 0.75g of protein per kilogram of body weight per day, although this will vary depending on activity levels[28].

Some people interested in gaining muscle weight choose to use protein supplements such as whey-based protein powders as there is some evidence this can increase muscle size when combined with weight-bearing exercise[29]. For most people this extra protein 'boost' is unnecessary as a balanced western diet typically contains more than enough protein. Adding more protein to your diet could even have a negative effect, as any protein consumed that is surplus to your body's requirements is likely to be stored as fat. On the other hand, insufficient protein intake can lead to muscle soreness and wastage, a lack of satiety (and possibly overeating to compensate!) and fatigue. Balanced consumption is the best way forward.

Where are they found? Protein is found in both animal and plant products. Meat, fish and other animal products such as eggs, cheese and milk contain high levels of protein, while plant-based sources include nuts, seeds, pulses and beans.

Different sources of protein? Veganism?

I'd recommend watching the film *Forks over Knives* for an insight into how we have come to believe that butter and cheese play a central role in an optimally healthy diet. Some see the film as vegan propaganda, but there is much contention about the supposed benefits and risks of a high-protein diet. For example, some studies suggest it is associated with a small increase in heart failure[30], while others suggest it helps heart patients live longer[31]. Overall the film has positive big messages showing how changing what you eat can do 'what medication has never done': reverse some medical conditions. But like all output with a message to promote (in this case veganism) there was a biased reporting of a study that implied that casein found in dairy products promotes cancer growth when consumed in large quantities.

I looked at the original study and it showed that those rats on a higher (20%) casein diet did develop cancer but they lived longer than those rats on a 5% casein diet[32]. So, in fact, whilst the latter were at lower risk of getting cancer, they died earlier, meaning those rats that had a protein deficiency and were far from healthy![33] I find this type of biased science-based reporting very disappointing.

One of the world's top cardiologists, Dr Joel Kahn, who has over 30 years of experience treating thousands of patients, has written *The Plant Based Solution* and he thinks these arguments are missing the point. He points out that B12 is a vitamin that cannot build up in the body at any toxic level and the fact that vegans may have to take it has become the soft underbelly for those who argue that a plant diet isn't optimal. The critics will say: "Well, you have to take supplements. How can that ever be an optimal diet?" He replies: "Well, yeah, you maybe take a B12 occasionally, a vitamin D, or an algae-based omega-3. But what *don't* you have to take? Insulin, statins, chemotherapy…" In fact, he would recommend B12 to all over 50s for optimal brain health, see Chapter 12 for more details on 'keeping your marbles'.

He says vegans can't claim total absence of disease. "I tell people eating plant diets to still follow medical guidelines because it enhances the odds of avoiding and reversing disease. It doesn't take them down to zero. So, the trade-off for one or two vitamins is an 80% reduction in the odds you're going to suffer chronic disease. I think most people would say that's a pretty good trade-off"[34].

However, if you do decide to get your protein from non-animal sources, you do have to consider the ways you can include calcium, omega-3 fatty acids, vitamin B12 and folate – key nutrients a vegan diet can lack. The RYG programme has a specific vegan course that addresses this potential imbalance.

So, what can we do as lay people? Eat a varied healthy diet whilst the experts battle it out!

Fruit and vegetables

Fruit and vegetables are the superstars of any balanced diet. In addition to providing plenty of fibre and vitamins, fruit and veg are also rich in polyphenols: key phytochemicals that reduce oxidative stress in your body by regulating the production of free radicals in your cells. Oxidative stress arises due to the presence of free radicals (highly reactive molecules produced in your body in response to exposure to pollutants), a compromised diet, smoking, and as a by-product of normal metabolism. Antioxidants occur naturally in foods and can decrease the number of free radicals in our body, but please see Chapter 13 for a full discussion on antioxidant supplementation and the distortion of scientific research for marketing purposes.

Fun fact: Polyphenols keep their stability when frozen, so frozen fruit and veg are still antioxidant rich.

Superfoods

When it comes to buzz words, 'superfoods' is right up there, but what exactly are they? There is no official definition, but they are broadly recognised as plant-based foods that are exceptionally rich in nutrients. I would say all good healthy food is a superfood! Below is a list of some truly 'super' fruits and vegetables.

Blueberries

- Contain anthocyanins, believed to have numerous health benefits including promoting cardiovascular health and protecting cells from free radicals which can be produced from natural metabolic processes[35].

- Their high fibre content helps to prevent constipation and, as we have seen, promote a healthy microbiome.

- Try it out: Start the day with blueberries in your yogurt, cereal, oatmeal or smoothie.

Broccoli

- High in vitamin C which helps to protect the body against viruses and infection[36]. In addition, its high vitamin K profile helps to strengthen bones thereby preventing bone fracture[37]. As a characteristic of cruciferous vegetables, broccoli contains sulforaphane that helps prevent colon cancer[38,39].

- Broccoli is considered one of the most powerful immunity-boosting foods, along with other vegetables in this cruciferous family (eg cabbage, cauliflower, turnip). It is high in sulphur-containing compounds, which are powerful stimulators of the immune system.

  Try it out: Add broccoli to stir-fry dishes or casseroles. An excellent side dish with most fish and meats.

Avocado

- Rich in several B vitamins (B1, B2, B3, B5, B6, and B9), folate, vitamins K, C and E.

- Contains lutein and zeaxanthin, which are important for eye health[40].

- Contains monounsaturated fats, which help to lower blood cholesterol levels[41].

  Try it out: Include avocado in your salad, smoothie, or as delicious guacamole.

Onions

- Contain a high level of quercetin, which is believed to help protect cells from free radical damage and they are a good prebiotic[42].

- Onions contain compounds which are thought to play roles in lowering blood pressure by helping to thin the blood, as well as reducing asthma symptoms and acting as natural antibiotics[43].

  Try it out: You can add onions to casseroles, pasta dishes and curries.

Observational studies have found that the consumption of nuts seems to have cancer preventative properties[44] when it comes to breast cancer and that it increases the survival rates of patients with colon cancer[45]. Mushrooms have also been shown to be anti-angiogenic (block cancer blood vessel growth), immune boosting and anti-inflammatory as they feed our healthy gut bacteria (the stem is especially full of goodness) and watercress has been shown to interfere with the activation of carcinogens that come from cigarette smoke[46].

So, which are the best?

Maybe don't worry about the details, just be sure to have lots of fresh vegetables and berries in your diet and make your plate colourful. Food and nutrition information on a piecemeal basis can be a distraction. Concentrate on the basics: fresh real food!

It may also be worth considering where you get your vegetables from and whether they've been doused in anything that might be bad for you. The Dirty Dozen and The Clean Fifteen refer to the fruits and vegetables that are typically the most and least contaminated by pesticides. The Dirty Dozen have been identified as containing particularly high quantities of pesticide residues when grown using conventional methods and are best bought organic. The Clean Fifteen, on the other hand, are less prone to contamination by pollutants, which makes them safer to be bought as non-organic.

Why organic? One argument is that it has more nutrients and the other is that it has less pesticide residue. Glyphosate used in many pesticides[47] acts as a chelator of good minerals and vitamins, actually reducing the availability of magnesium and inactivating vitamin D.

Too expensive? Ask yourself what is the real cost of eating non-organic food? I would go on record as saying that following the Dirty Dozen, Clean Fifteen explained below) over a lifetime could prevent bad health that you may have because of a compromised diet. We must as far as possible vote with our wallets to save our gut bacteria and our planet.

The exact products on these lists change quite frequently and I am aware that organic systems vary along with the fertility of the soil, but you can still use them as a guide to help you make informed choices next time you visit the supermarket.

The Dirty Dozen

1. Strawberries
2. Spinach
3. Nectarines
4. Apples
5. Peaches
6. Pears
7. Cherries
8. Grapes
9. Celery
10. Tomatoes and lettuce
11. Sweet bell peppers
12. Potatoes

The Clean Fifteen

1. Sweetcorn and sweet potatoes
2. Avocados
3. Pineapples
4. Cabbage
5. Onions
6. Peas
7. Papayas
8. Asparagus
9. Mangos
10. Aubergine
11. Honeydew melon
12. Kiwi
13. Cantaloupe melon
14. Cauliflower
15. Grapefruit

The RYG programme has been carefully designed to take account of these lists and to use readily available and economic ingredients.

In a paper entitled 'The Power of Functional Nutrition' by the Institute for Functional Medicine on their website they state that when high-quality nutrition is "applied effectively and consistently" it can prevent chronic disease[48], enhance cognition in people with dementia[49], and amongst other things improve surgical recovery[50]. This to me seems to make sense and I would encourage you to eat well to support your general health as well as prevent and reverse chronic diseases.

Summing up

- Eat plenty of natural wholefoods

- Avoid processed foods

- Reduce your intake of refined sugars

- Limit your intake of saturated fats

- Increase your intake of nutrient-rich fruit and vegetables (see Chapter 13 for more on specific vitamins and minerals)

- Consider doing the RYG online programme to ensure you know which foods are gut friendly

- High-quality nutrition is essential to prevent and reverse chronic diseases

Notes:

Notes:

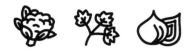

CHAPTER 3

Exercise

Research from Cambridge University recently showed that lack of exercise is theoretically twice as likely to kill you as being obese[1]. And if that doesn't have you reaching for your trainers, a report published in *The Lancet* warned that being sedentary is just as bad for your heart as smoking a packet of cigarettes a day. Lack of exercise is the new smoking in terms of health risks.

Being active, as you will see in this book, is not only proven to lower the risk of heart disease, type 2 diabetes, stroke[2], osteoporosis and various cancers, it also keeps your weight under control, improves sleep, helps with stress, anxiety and depression[3] and may even help you to live longer. Researchers have also found that loss of leg muscle is associated with slower walking speeds[4] and this is linked to a lower 10-year survival rate for people after 75[5].

You don't need to pump iron for hours on end or run marathons to be fit (though obviously that's fine for people who have the time and stamina!). Exercise can still be easily incorporated into your life to help your body and mind stay healthy. Try to keep it regular to get into a habit yet varied enough to keep it interesting. Find something you love, and you will do it. Make it a challenge or social. Whatever floats your boat. Let's have a look at what you could be doing and why exercise is so good for you.

How your body and mind benefit from exercise

Increasing your lifespan and keeping quality of life

Studies have shown that keeping active is key for you to have a longer and healthier and more rewarding life[6], after all, no one really wants to get old and be constantly unwell. One research project involving 6,600 participants revealed that people who increased their activity levels to 150 minutes a week (the amount recommended by the World Health Organisation [WHO]) saw their predicted life expectancy rise by more than three years[7].

Muscles

As you get older, your muscle density shrinks, making you more vulnerable to injuries, aches and falls. Regular resistance exercise (at least twice a week, see description below) can help you to increase muscle strength, as well as boosting your balance. It can also improve your sleep and posture and increase your metabolic rate. There is evidence to suggest that resistance training can improve blood glucose controls for diabetics, reduce pain in people with rheumatoid arthritis and reduce the risk of osteoporosis[8–10].

The best way for you to increase muscle strength is with weights, squats and press-ups. To improve muscle endurance, which is your body's ability to sustain low to moderate exercise over an extended period, it is best to try running or swimming. Yoga and martial arts can increase your flexibility – your ability to move joints effectively through a range of motions.

Bone strength

When you think about exercising, keeping your heart healthy and your body strong are probably the pay-offs you are most focused on. But maintaining bone density is also important, especially as you get older.

Bone is a living tissue that responds to increases in loads by getting stronger, as movement causes muscles to pull on the bones they are anchored to by tendons. Weight itself increases the loading capacity of the skeleton, which is why being too thin can lead to weaker bones.

According to the National Osteoporosis Society (nos.org.uk), weight-bearing exercises, like jogging or dancing, are best for increasing bone strength. Research has shown that in tennis, considered a high-intensity sport, players have greater bone density in their dominant serving arm compared to their non-serving arm[11].

Luckily, bone strength is something we can all improve on; scientists at Loughborough University revealed that men over 65 who started hopping for just two minutes a day were able to significantly increase both bone density and strength[12].

Microbes

The microbiome is still an emerging area of health. The research on the link between gut bacteria and exercise is largely limited to studies on mice and rats, but there is evidence to suggest that regularly working out helps to encourage good microbial balance in the gut[13,14]. In my practice I encourage clients to get enough sleep and exercise in addition to eating well for the maximum diversity in their gut bacteria, and as you have read in Chapter 1, increased diversity of the microbiome has many positive effects on your body.

Heart

In the UK, someone suffers a heart attack every three minutes. Cardiovascular disease remains the world's biggest killer, responsible for 26% of all deaths[15]. A policy paper released by the UK Department of Health reveals that a quarter of all fatal heart attacks occur in people under the age of 75, and many of these deaths could be preventable[16].

Apart from lowering your cholesterol and trying to stick to a largely plant-based Mediterranean diet, being active can reduce the body's resistance to insulin, reducing your chances of developing type 2 diabetes. Insulin resistance promotes inflammation[17] – which is also linked to heart disease.

According to the British Heart Foundation, regular exercise can help to reduce your risk of heart disease by up to 35%[18]. Exercise can also lower your resting heart rate and blood pressure, further reducing your risk of cardiovascular disorders[19].

Doing 150 minutes of moderate-intensity exercise a week will help to keep your heart healthy. This is the kind of exercise that makes you sweat and gets your heart beating faster – think cycling or fast walking.

Sleep

I'm sure everyone can relate to feeling exhausted after a long day of being physical – perhaps after redecorating a room in your house or digging the garden – and then you sleep 'like a log'. It should come as no surprise that exercise has proven to be beneficial for those suffering with common sleep disorders such as insomnia and obstructive sleep apnoea[20–22].

Sex

Diminishing sexual function is often dismissed as a natural part of ageing. It's worth noting, however, that regular exercise has been shown to improve sexual function in both men and women. Studies have reported that exercise generally improves sexual function[2], more specifically in males with chronic heart issues[25] and in females taking antidepressants[23] and with stress incontinence[24]. Please see Chapter 6 for more recent research on preventing erectile dysfunction.

Exercise boosts the brain

Memory

Generally, if something is good for your heart, it is likely to have a positive effect on your brain too. Various studies have shown that the hippocampus, an area of the brain heavily implicated in memory and learning, increases in volume in response to regular aerobic exercise[26,27]. Research from Germany showed that cycling whilst learning a foreign language led to significantly better retention of vocabulary[28,29].

Exam results

In Naperville, Arizona, gym teachers conducted an educational experiment called 'Zero Hour PE'. They scheduled time for the pupils to work out before class using treadmills and other exercise equipment and competing against themselves to improve.

In 1999, students from Naperville eighth grade took an international test known as TIMSS (Trends in International Mathematics and Science Study). They finished sixth in maths and first in science – an astonishing feat as in the previous years students from China, Japan and Singapore had always finished ahead.

The programme turned the 19,000 students into not only some of the fittest in the USA but also, in some categories, the 'smartest in the world'!

An innovative maths teacher at Great Marlow School, Buckinghamshire, who also runs the rowing squad, was fed up with fielding questions from parents about the amount of time training took out of their children's study time, so he decided to do the maths. Inspired by reading the Naperville story in the book *Spark* by Dr John Ratey, he collected data over four years to compare how his rowers' academic results stacked up against the school in general. Game, set, pull: the rowers consistently outperformed their cohort academically.

High-intensity training for any team or individual sport will raise the need to look at consumption of carbohydrates before the sport so that the carbs that are stored as glycogen in our muscles can be used as an energy source rather than the body drawing on the muscles for energy and causing muscle wastage.

Concentration

I realise that some people may require a randomised control trial to really believe exercise can help the brain. Here it is.

In 2014, researchers at the University of Illinois demonstrated that being fit can lead to better focus. The study involved 211 children, aged between seven and nine, who spent nine months at an hour-long after-school exercise programme. When the programme was over, the researchers found that the children involved showed widespread changes in brain function, and were far more effective at blocking out distractions than their classmates who weren't on the programme[30].

There is also evidence to suggest that short bursts of exercise may have a positive impact on ADHD. A study involving 32 men with ADHD revealed that the participants were more energetic and motivated to complete a given task after a vigorous 20-minute bike ride[31].

Prevents cognitive decline

Did you know that exercise can change the structure of your brain and help to kick-start the parts that aren't working as well? This process of creating new pathways in the brain is known as neuroplasticity. Regular exercise can help produce chemicals that contribute to the formation of new neural connections. If you're worried about losing your marbles as you get older, then you should know that, according to researchers at the University of Cambridge[32], just doing one hour of vigorous exercise a week can halve your risk of developing Alzheimer's disease, and a study by scientists at UCLA reported three changes in the brain when people exercise[33]:

- The size of the brain's memory centre increases

- Memory performance improves

- Brain Derived Neurotrophic Factor (BDNF) levels go up, which stimulates the growth of new brain cells

Laura Farey, a personal trainer, reports how getting 93-year-old Fred, who was sedentary and not speaking, walking every day changed his mental state almost instantly. He went from an old man with dementia sitting in a chair, to speaking animatedly about his past life and taking an interest in his food. The power of exercise is immense at any age.

Mental health

Moving your body releases a cascade of hormones with positive effects on your body and mind. Exercise makes you feel great and serves as an excellent way to ward off depression and low moods. Getting physically fit and achieving personal goals can boost your self-esteem, and if you work out in a group or with friends it's a great way to socialise.

A young man I worked with, let's call him Thomas, was having panic attacks and, from the age of 15, refused to go to school. He was gay and bullied by some of his classmates. He had low self-esteem, low moods, was gaining weight and had made several suicide attempts and self-harmed. Talking therapy CBT (see Chapter 5) has shown that behavioural activation is an effective intervention on its own for depression[35,36], but to further aid recovery I suggested a one-off personal training session, followed by an exercise app of his own choice to encourage exercise on a regular basis. He is now slim, confident and enjoying life.

Farey worked with a lady aged 35 who was seriously depressed and had lost her job. Farey explains: "After a few 1:1 trainings and regular workouts, she found a new job, lost five stone and came off all medication." We all know these stories and often, because of the constraints of low income and family demands, it can be a case of needing motivating to start. There are many exercise apps that can be the motivation which would be cheaper than a personal trainer; take the time to find one that suits you.

Exercise builds resilience to stress

When we are stressed, our bodies release cortisol and adrenaline, which not only interfere with appetite but also leave our brains feeling fuzzy. Being under stress, especially chronic stress, can make it more difficult to find the time and energy to be physically active[37]. It is ironic, perhaps, that exercise is one of the best ways to deal with stress. If you've ever gone for a run to escape from deadlines or dilemmas, you've probably returned feeling calmer and more able to cope. Exercise helps to reduce the level of stress hormones and stimulates the production of endorphins, the body's natural mood elevators. Mindfulness exercises such as those taught in yoga have been shown to reduce stimulation of the amygdala, an area of the brain involved in emotions such as stress and anxiety[38].

Activity makes you happier

There really is such a thing as the 'runner's high'. Exercise is like a natural antidepressant as it triggers the release of our 'happy hormones', serotonin and dopamine. In fact, many doctors now encourage patients with mild depression and anxiety to join a gym. In one German study, clinically depressed participants were asked to walk quickly on a treadmill for 30 minutes a day over a 10-day period. At the end of the experiment, researchers recorded a significant drop in depression scores[39]. It has, in fact, long been proven that people scored higher for mood, memory and energy, and lower for depression, tension and anxiety after physical exercise[40].

How much?

The World Health Organisation recommends 150 minutes (2.5 hours) of moderate exercise or 75 minutes (1 hour 15 minutes) of vigorous exercise per week[41] and this is potentially able to extend your lifespan[42].

Some what I view as extreme exercise research has shown that the greatest health gains occur after six hours of vigorous exercise or 12 hours of moderate exercise per week. Increasing activity to these levels reduced the risk of heart disease, stroke, colon cancer and diabetes by around 20% and breast cancer by 6%[43].

This does seem to me quite difficult to fit into our busy modern lives, and as one wise physiotherapist said to me: "It would all have to be done with an eye on injury prevention otherwise the end result could be no exercise at all for a while!"

I think the best approach is always to take the middle line. If you include walking in moderate exercise and aim for five hours of moderate exercise per week, this to me feels manageable. It up to you, do what works for you, but one thing is clear: you have to do some!

When to exercise

Some people prefer to exercise bright and early, before the day begins; others prefer to work out after work or in the evenings. Really, the best time to exercise is when you feel like it. A functional test that I do with clients looks at an individual's genetics and what is the best time and type of exercise (see Chapter 11). So, if you are looking to achieve a record time or a personal best, look at your genetics first (but always try to consult a certified genetic counsellor).

Keep moving

In our modern office-bound world, we can spend upwards of seven hours sitting each day, which studies have suggested is associated with early mortality[45]. Studies have linked such inactivity to type 2 diabetes, obesity and various cardiovascular diseases[46]. In fact, the World Health Organisation lists inactivity as the fourth greatest factor contributing to premature death. Indeed, the American Medical Association is so concerned by the amount of time we spend sitting that they issued a recommendation that companies should provide their employees with standing or treadmill desks[47].

If you do spend a lot of time stuck at a desk (and let's face it, most of us do) make sure you get out for a brisk walk every day. Around 20 minutes of walking a day (roughly 150 minutes a week) can cut your risk of heart disease and stroke; it will also clear your head and give you a break from your demon computer!

Getting moving is especially important if you have had an operation. Laura Farey, the personal trainer mentioned earlier, tells a story of Rosita who had a hip replacement. After concentrating on regaining fitness, Rosita was able to ride competitively again. I myself have had a ruptured anterior crucial ligament in my knee and underwent innovative surgery involving stem cell, extracted from a cadaver, to repair my mashed cartilage and hamstring, and replace my torn ligament. I then started a structured daily physiotherapy programme.

It is important to maintain sufficient muscle mass as, depending on your fitness levels, the body can start to lose muscle after just two to three days. I used a Compex machine to help me during the two weeks after my operation, which allowed me to do the equivalent of 100 squats without getting out of bed. These machines are used by top athletes to maintain muscle mass after injury. My knee at the age of 56 is good to go, but only because I kept moving and did not lose any muscle mass.

Well worth remembering that keeping moving will help you to have a healthier body as well as a happier mind.

Types of exercise

Get sweaty

No matter what time of day you decide to work out and how often, the important thing is to sweat. Perspiring helps us to regulate our body temperature by allowing evaporative cooling. Sweat is made up of mostly water, but also contains antimicrobial peptides such as dermcidin, which are effective in fighting off viruses, fungi and damaging bacteria. These peptides target the cell membranes of bacteria, and show promise for use in the development of treatments for bacterial conditions that are resistant to conventional antibiotic treatments[44].

Aerobic exercise

This kind of exercise helps to speed up your heart and breathing rate, giving your heart and lungs a good workout. It can also lower blood sugar levels, 'bad' LDL cholesterol and blood pressure whilst burning fat and reducing inflammation.

What to do: Running, swimming, jogging, dancing and many exercise classes such as aerobics.

Why not try? High Intensity Interval Training (HIIT) is a relatively new form of exercise which typically lasts for 20 minutes and involves pushing yourself as hard as you can for 30 seconds before resting for 20 seconds and then repeating. Because these sessions are so much shorter than standard exercise classes, some people assume they are easier, but trainers warn that this really isn't the case – you will feel your muscles ache afterwards!

HIIT isn't the ideal class if you have underlying health problems and poor fitness levels as it is very strenuous. HIIT training has been shown to reduce blood sugar levels, in addition to improving endurance, strength and muscle tone, but research has also shown that more accessible, moderate regimes following the interval training pattern of exercise and recovery (see below) can have beneficial effects on cardiovascular fitness[48,49].

Interval walking

If you fancy something a little less arduous, you can't go far wrong with interval walking, which has been used for decades as a training method by elite athletes. Simply alternate bursts of moderate walking with shorter stints of much brisker walking, perhaps walking gently for 100 steps and then fast for 50.

Resistance exercise

Regular strength training and weight bearing improves your strength, posture and balance and helps to keep your bones and muscles healthy.

What to do: Try yoga, Pilates, weight lifting, squats or sit-ups. If you're not keen on the gym, carrying shopping, heavier housework chores and gardening can also help to build strength. In fact, mowing the lawn – using a push mower, not a ride-on – burns more calories than playing badminton. Pilates or yoga challenge your flexibility, balance, core fitness and strength. Walking is a great weight-bearing exercise for your legs!

Why not try? The plank – this is an easy resistance exercise which improves core strength. Simply lie on your front and raise your body up on to your toes and hands, bringing your hips and shoulders level (as if you were about to do a press-up). Hold this pose for ten seconds before releasing down on to your knees for ten seconds. Repeat ten times, increasing the time you hold the pose as you are able.

Balance exercise

When it comes to good balance, it really is a case of 'use it or lose it' – especially as we get older. Our sense of balance is controlled by the vestibular system, an intricate collection of tubes and chambers in the inner ear, which becomes less effective in most people over the age of 55.

Having good core strength and balance is particularly important for older people, as according to the Centre for Ageing Better, 30% of people over the age of 65 will have a fall every year, which can result in severe injury. Annually, there are 250,000 emergency hospital admissions in the UK due to falls or fractures[50].

Note: Fractures can be due to osteoporosis, a loss in bone mineral density that weakens the bones making them more fragile and more likely to break, which affects over 3 million people in the UK according to the NHS. Weight-bearing exercises are crucial to strengthen your bones – try standing on one leg while brushing your teeth as a start! In a well-designed placebo-controlled study, probiotics were also shown to reduce the rate of bone loss in the elderly. The study suggests that what we eat can help prevent osteoporosis with probiotics, as well as exercise[51].

What to do: Golf, fencing, gymnastics, yoga or lawn bowls.

Why not try? Tai chi – originally from China and often described as 'meditation in motion', this mind-body practice has many recognised health benefits. Tai chi is safe, low impact and relaxing. Tai chi not only boosts balance but also increases the body's strength and flexibility.

The human body is naturally designed to be active, as you will see in the conclusion of the book; in communities where people regularly live to 100+ they are regularly physically active. It is not natural for us to sit all day!

Summing up

- Regular exercise throughout your week can extend your life by protecting you from ill-health and disease, giving you a better quality, longer lifespan

- Mixing it up can benefit different parts of your body as muscles need to be in balance

- Regular exercise benefits your brain and mental health as well as your physical body

- Regular activity improves memory and focus and makes you feel good

- Aim for a mixture of aerobic, resistance and balance to keep it fun and interesting

Notes:

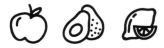

CHAPTER 4

Mental health

Patients suffering from mental health problems are often encouraged to process and 'think' their way out of their current mental state and to use the power of thought coupled with talking therapies to alleviate their depression and anxiety. What isn't considered in such an approach is the physical aspect of mental health problems, for example a compromised microbiome or a low vitamin D level.

This may sound like I am arguing against my own work – yes and no. I have found through clinical experience that talking therapies have their place, *but* they are so much more powerful when combined with paying attention to physical aspects of a person too. The end results for the patient are often more permanent and life enhancing.

When your brain is in a healthy state you can enjoy life to the fullest, it means your amazing sensory capabilities can be fully enjoyed. Your sense of taste, ability to smell, see and hear all rely on you having a healthy nervous system, through which electrical signals are transmitted to your brain. When your brain function is compromised by your physiology, brought on by bad nutrition, poor exercise and stressful environments, mental health problems such as burning out and fatigue can occur. Mental and physical health are inextricably linked, and a pill for one will not cure the other!

What affects our brains?

I have had clients who really struggle with the concept that the brain is directly affected by what we put in our mouth and who do not understand the correlation between their quality of life with their food choices. When these doubting clients make the sometimes reluctant effort to pay attention to the vitamins, minerals and phytochemicals in what they eat, the results are nothing short of miraculous.

Rebecca, a client complaining of brain fog and lack of energy, felt she was on energy levels of 110% within four weeks of the RYG programme. The brain is hugely vulnerable to negative nutritional input; it requires balanced nutritional input to help clear out waste products from the normal metabolic processes in the brain. If your diet is deficient in key micronutrients, your brain cannot function in a normal way.

To have a happy brain you must have good communication between the gut and the brain, but this is often disturbed by an imbalance of chemicals in the system, perhaps caused by stress or what we are eating. As you read in Chapter 1, research shows that microbial diversity is essential to a fully functioning brain, and it has been shown that the intestines have an incredible network for exchanging biochemicals with the brain. We will see in this chapter that emerging research shows that when the microbiome is well balanced, it can communicate with the brain correctly and that this, in turn, helps with mental health challenges[1].

Studies have linked leaky gut with irritable bowel syndrome (IBS) and it affects 10-15% of the population, but in both major depressive and general anxiety disorders it is found at a higher rate of 25%[2]. Dr Kellman, in *The Whole Brain Diet*, looks at a healthy microbiome being a solution to "healing depression, anxiety and brain fog without prescription drugs". He suggests that a leaky gut alters the microbiome, which in turn leads to an inflammatory state (see Chapter 6). This then cues the central nervous system towards depression and other cognitive disorders.

The RYG programme is designed to help heal a leaky gut by introducing gut-healing foods, and with the figures above showing the incidence of IBS is up to 15% higher in people with mental health conditions, this approach must be crucial in aiding recovery.

In *Fast Food Genocide*, Dr Joel Fuhrman cites compelling evidence that excessive consumption of processed food and fizzy drinks is contributing to a myriad of physical health problems as well as lowering our intelligence, fostering antisocial behaviour and creating mental illness. He states that the human brain is sensitive to nutritional input, resulting in mental health conditions and non-diagnosable problems such as negative thinking, anger, loss of mental clarity and violence to self or others.

Dr Sarah McKay states further that there is "a clear relationship between diet and the level of mental health, especially in young people" and is excited that "we're right at the dawn of a whole new way of thinking about brain development and brain health. And the neuroscientific evidence for the role of the microbiome is just getting stronger and stronger at the basic level"[3]. A poor diet puts people in this prison and they cannot see a way out, so end up going to doctors for medication rather than fixing the issue themselves.

It is my choice what I eat!

Personally, I get it when people push back and say to me it is their choice to eat badly. Indeed, I believe life is about your freedom of choice. However, there is one thing that bothers me about this approach. For example, with fast foods so high in sugar that is absorbed so quickly into your bloodstream and stimulates your pleasurable dopamine receptors in the brain, how much choice do you really have? In fact, after a while the brain becomes dopamine insensitive and you will need more sugary food to get the same degree of pleasure. You may become overweight and possibly develop a mental health issue. Did you choose that?

It is a fact that major food companies hire neuroscientists to identify the 'bliss point', using MRI scans to figure out what combination of additives and flavourings would ensure that consumers would struggle to stop ingesting the chosen food[4]. A flavour that explodes in your mouth and then implodes your gut bacteria! They combine fat, sugar and salt to create a perfect taste known in the industry as the 'bliss point', which is totally addictive. Does that mean you are choosing to eat it?

Whilst the research on this area is developing, the evidence on the 'rock face' of therapy is compelling: unhealthy eating is fuelling a spiral of depression and anxiety. Researchers are looking for which bacteria affects your mental health with the aim of either "modifying those bacteria, putting in more beneficial bacteria or reducing harmful bacteria" in the hope "that this might be a way to see improved behaviour"[5].

It is essential to avoid inflammatory foods and to guard against deficiencies of B12, magnesium, zinc and fatty acids, all of which are essential for energy and mood regulation. In my practice, I have seen people recover their health, lose weight, get rid of diabetes and come off antidepressants and other drugs by paying attention to what they are putting in their mouths. (The RYG programme is a way of starting this process.)

The status quo

Currently mainstream mental health treatments are also being held back by the requirement for a diagnosis via the Diagnostic and Statistical Manual of Mental Disorders (DSM). The definition of mental illnesses in the DSM can be imprecise and is sometimes defined in the context of brain areas or the presence of certain biochemicals or list of behaviours.

Dr Chatterjee, a leading functional medicine practitioner, says he started to go down the functional health route as he felt he wasn't seeing "the whole person". One day he saw a young woman with depression. "My guidance (from the DSM and drug bibles) suggested I should prescribe her antidepressants but I felt this was wrong. She needed to talk." He saw her twice a week and let her talk and "we got her better".

Dr Ruth Baer, in her book *Practising Happiness*, highlights how the DSM is adding more and more disorders, and there are many overlaps. It is impossible for a therapist to learn them all. She suggests it would be better to have a transdiagnostic approach that is more integrative, including relaxation techniques, cognitive destructing, psycho education, exposure and behavioural interventions, looking at patients' strengths and maximise purpose with meditation to increase positive emotion[6].

This is all good stuff and progress, but in my view separating the mental from the physical is meaningless; the client is best viewed as a complete and complex organism[1]. A very successful approach is to address your compromised microbiome in combination with a talking therapy of your choice: see www.maphealthsolutions.com.

The DSM does not consider whether a client has a compromised gut microbiome or what a patient is eating. It may well be that the current research, in many cases funded by the pharmaceutical companies, or driven by academics who are passionate about their area of talking therapies, has not caught up with this new area of functional mental health. There is one study that aimed to see if the talking therapy Cognitive Behavioural Therapy (CBT) could help with irritable bowel syndrome, but overwhelming diagnoses for mental health conditions are separated from the physical body condition, and this is worse than meaningless[1].

A study in the *Journal of the American Academy of Child and Adolescent Psychiatry* reported that established treatments for chronic depression and anxiety such as SSRI antidepressants and CBT were only effective in the long term for 22% of patients. They took a cohort of 319 teenagers, and whilst around 48% reported an initial improvement, after six years this reduced to just 22%.

The difference between being free of anxiety and depression, or not, could be strongly associated with family support and the absence of 'negative life events'. However, I would suggest that had they looked at the whole cohort and accessed data on nutritional deficiencies, sleep patterns, exercise and then sought to address the physical at the same time as the mental, the rate of success would be far higher than 22%, which has to be a very disappointing result for any therapeutic approach[7].

So before committing to a course of medication or talking therapy, please consider looking into other physical issues that may underlie your problems.

The future

Sadly, many of us, at least to some degree, are 'wounded soldiers'[1] and will suffer from anxiety, depression, brain fog, memory issues, lack of motivation, difficulty in focusing, making intellectual connections, accomplishing tasks, learning, feeling stuck, the world is grey, irritable, and have sleep issues at some time in our lives. In the case of traumatic incidences such as divorce, loss of a loved one, redundancy, and dealing with debt, talking therapies are amazing at unravelling the damage and decreasing the stress caused. However, yet again here, I would suggest this would be even more successful if it was combined with a functional mental health approach which can address the accompanying symptoms of poor brain function.

I would also apply this to all other therapies and disciplines such as chiropractic therapy, physiotherapy, reflexology, mainstream or holistic, evidenced based or placebo. They may all make a difference but would make so much more of a difference if done in conjunction with the client, checking out their physical state, checking out their microbiome, improving their nutrition, exercising and relaxing.

In my view, nutritional psychiatry is the future of mental health treatment.

Studies are showing for example that in first episode psychosis patients (pre-drug treatment), their microbiome was different from that of the healthy matched control individuals[8]. In other words, the microbiome was compromised. The hypothesis is, because of the gut-brain connection, this may have contributed to the mental health problem occurring.

A Harvard Health Blog reported in 2018[9] that "on average, the reduction in readmission was 74% lower in the probiotic combination compared with the placebo arm of the study. The most significant finding was an almost 90% reduction of hospitalisation in the group with the highest inflammation score who took probiotics". In other words, there was a significantly lower bipolar readmission rate for the group taking probiotics compared to the control, and this suggests that gut bacteria is related to being bipolar.

This approach that gut health does affect mental health is not widely accepted by mainstream medicine yet, but a lack of essential nutrients has been thought to contribute to poor mental health[10] including conditions such as anxiety, depression, bipolar disorder, schizophrenia and ADHD.

The NICE (National Institute for Health and Care Excellence) guidelines in the UK only recommend talking therapies and antidepressants. This is a big disconnect with reality. Many mental health conditions are, at least in part, caused by inflammation in the brain, and this could start in our gut due to deficiencies in key nutrients such as magnesium, omega-3 fatty acids, probiotics, vitamins and minerals.

For example, in one study a magnesium citrate supplement led to a significant improvement in depression and anxiety, regardless of age, gender or severity of depression. The improvement did not continue when the supplement was stopped[11]. Patients who were given 248mg of magnesium per day (with vitamin B6 that is required to absorb it) had reversed their depressive symptoms, and this approach was at least 10 pence per day cheaper than prescription drugs[12]!

The study stated: "The results are very encouraging, given the great need for additional treatment options for depression, and our finding that magnesium supplementation provides a safe, fast and inexpensive approach to controlling depressive symptoms." They emphasised that good nutrition is an important contributor to mental health, but it is clear in some cases that supplementation would not be able to replace antidepressants altogether and it is wise to always consult your GP before coming off antidepressants.

So if you find it hard to believe that improving the balance of your microbiome and nutritional intake will help your mental health, why not get tested, see a nutritionist, reset your gut and see how you feel. It can do no harm.

If you think this option is an expensive one, then just look at changing the way you eat via the RYG programme as you must buy food anyway. People who take this route are finding it either cheaper as they are buying less meat or at the most up to 20% more expensive per week when they are doing the reset. I have had clients on very low incomes undertake the RYG programme and become experts at ensuring they are at local markets when the stallholders are packing up so they can buy fruit and vegetables at knock-down prices.

There is a direct connection between food, inflammation and mental illness. Mainstream medical doctors have little nutritional knowledge as it is traditionally excluded from medical degrees. However, the evidence is mounting and for the sake of our mental health we must take nutrition seriously.

I had one client, Martin, who diagnostically had been told he had 'chronic long-term depression'. He made dramatic improvements within three weeks of starting the RYG programme and a daily morning walk. His tested levels of depression after these three weeks were sub-clinical (ie showing very few symptoms).

If you are taking medications it will require medical supervision to reduce the dose as they affect the function of your brain, but if you are not taking medications I would encourage you to do the RYG programme first.

Clients of mine who have committed to resetting their gut along with the talking therapies detailed in Chapter 5 have had enormous shifts. They have found new passions, or dropped unwanted habits, and their anxiety and depression has lifted. It is no less than transformative. By fully considering the impact of the environment and lifestyle on their bodies, and more particularly their microbiome, they say things like "I have got *me* back" and "I have my drive again." Fab!

Personally, a few years ago I was faced with a mental health challenge, and at first I did not realise what was wrong. I went to see various doctors and on three occasions they tried to prescribe me antidepressants. I knew I was not depressed. After a traumatic event involving one of my children, I started losing weight, not eating properly, avoiding social situations, and became fearful of similar situations arising. I trusted no one and even reading about a similar event would make me have unpleasant side effects.

Eventually a wonderful local GP called Dr Williams sat and listened to my list of symptoms. He recognised that I was not going to take the drugs out of choice and that I was not depressed. He said I had 80% of the symptoms of PTSD. As soon as I sought professional help via CBT and other interventions I was able to start recovery. I also started eating well, exercising and reaching out to friends again.

The positive side of this experience was that I learned to surround myself with people who see the good in others (I find unkindness very difficult to deal with) and, whilst I still have flashbacks, I know that the lifestyle changes I made and having great friends is the best antidote to prevent the symptoms impacting my life.

This experience has massively informed my clinical practice and I always encourage clients to look at lifestyle changes to support their mental health recovery. In a very direct way it has brought me to designing the RYG programme, as I have seen that paying attention to the physical side of your health has a direct impact on your mental health, whether you are taking a drug to help you or not.

Mental illnesses

Depression

There is now growing awareness that depression is a serious illness, not simply an inability to cope with everyday life. Notable world leaders like Winston Churchill, Abraham Lincoln and Mahatma Gandhi all suffered from depression, and according to data compiled by NHS Choices, one in ten of us will experience it at some point.

Symptoms of depression include tearfulness, a lack of appetite or overeating, an inability to sleep, irritability, difficulty making decisions, and extreme feelings of guilt, sadness and hopelessness[13]. Sufferers typically start to struggle at work and begin to avoid social events and activities they'd normally enjoy.

The causes of depression are varied, and some people develop 'reactive' depression after stressful life events such as bereavement, divorce, redundancy and even having a baby. In others, depression may be due to overwork, illness, social isolation, or nutritional and hormonal imbalances. It can also be a side effect of prescription drugs or, as discussed, a lack of diversity in your microbiome.

Although women are twice as likely to suffer from depression, men are more vulnerable to suicide as they are less likely to ask for help. Recent data from the Organisation of Economic Cooperation and Development revealed that one in ten Europeans were depressed, with 11% of British women and 8% of men claiming to be suffering from depression to some degree or another.

Studies have shown that variations in the serotonin transporter gene, which affects serotonin transport in the brain, can determine how we respond to stressful life events. People who have a variable sequence at the beginning of the gene which is 'short' are more likely to be diagnosed with depressive symptoms and suicidal feelings[14]. It is possible to test for your genetic predisposition to some mental health challenges (see Chapter 11 and www.maphealthsolutions.com).

But even though there is evidence that depression can be inherited[15], there are variables that will affect whether you actually end up developing depression. A lot can depend on the environmental factors, so even if you have family members with a history of depression, it doesn't mean you're doomed and you should just give up. Quite the opposite, it should encourage you to be more proactive and do everything in your power to prevent depression by paying attention to your nutrition and lifestyle.

Popular antidepressants like Prozac can effectively alleviate depression for some people but don't work on everyone[16] and their effects are not shown to last[17]. They also do not address the cause of the illness. The theory originating from the 1950s suggesting that low levels of serotonin are to blame for depression is now losing scientific credibility[18], as researchers found that individuals with low serotonin do not necessarily develop depressive symptoms, and that some antidepressants increase serotonin while others decrease it or have no serotonergic effect at all[19]. This study also seems to suggest that antidepressants are only effective for those with notable chemical imbalances in the brain.

Edward Bullmore, head of psychiatry at the University of Cambridge, theorises that mental health issues really do seem to be linked to the immune system and inflammation. In a 2017 study by the Department of Psychiatry in Cambridge, it was found that anti-inflammatory medicine may alleviate the symptoms of depression[20]. They looked at previous studies that showed patients with depression tend to experience inflammation[21] and have higher amounts of inflammatory cytokines (inflammation-causing proteins) in their blood[22,23].

This research is exciting as it may lead to a reduction in the inappropriate use of traditional antidepressants. However, researchers are still looking for a drug-based solution. I would suggest doctors and patients look at non-drug methods to reduce inflammation first like the RYG programme. Of course, for the patient, this will take more effort as it is not a simple pill but a lifestyle change that could include:

- Walk or run for 30 minutes a day

- Cut out sugar[24] and sweeteners

- Eat fresh, natural, inflammation-fighting food[25]

- Drink coffee in moderation (see Chapter 7)[26] and less alcohol[27]

- Get seven hours sleep a night[28]

- Practise meditation and mindfulness[29]

- Surround yourself with family and friends[30]

- Get a sense of purpose[31]

- And of course do the *Reset Your Gut* programme, which is rich in all the minerals and vitamins and other nutritional requirements for good mental health

I researched the above papers in detail, and none of these will treat depression on its own. Some have evidence from rats, and others like mindfulness had a 'small to moderate effect'; however I would suggest that combined they would definitely be worth a try to avoid taking a drug with side effects.

Note: As you will see discussed in Chapter 7, finding a cure is not in the drug industries' best interests, it affects their bottom line. In the USA alone, 254 million prescriptions for antidepressants are written every year at a cost of $10bn[32].

Anxiety

It is perfectly normal to feel anxious from time to time, but people with anxiety disorders have an exaggerated and often chronic response to worry. This can cause a whole range of physical effects, from poor appetite to insomnia, digestive issues, and a racing heart, as well as feelings of intense panic and fear. There is no doubt that anxiety can be an incredibly debilitating condition with many sufferers cutting themselves off and avoiding situations that may trigger an anxiety attack.

A study from the University of Oxford has recently shown in healthy volunteers that a prebiotic intervention can increase one's attention to positive stimuli, a proxy marker for optimism[33], clearly implicating that our gut impacts our mood. The same groups have also shown that the same prebiotic substance can decrease anxiety and improve cognitive function[34], based on trials in rats. In mice, research has shown a gut-brain connection[35] and that the ingestion of probiotics affects the balance of the microbiome and plays an important role in regulating emotional behaviour. The RYG programme includes both pre- and probiotics for humans.

From an economic perspective, a study compiled by researchers from the University of Cambridge and the University of Hertfordshire revealed that 18.7% of the UK population suffered from anxiety to some degree in 2010, costing the British economy about £10bn a year[36].

According to the charity Anxiety UK, one in ten people will develop a debilitating anxiety disorder. Symptoms can begin at any stage of life, and women are twice as likely to suffer from anxiety as men. It is believed that an area of the brain called the amygdala, which is involved in feelings of fear and danger, is more reactive in people with anxiety[37,38]. I have found that EFT (see Chapter 5) is particularly effective as a self-help approach to reducing anxiety in my clients.

Eating disorders

Although not as prevalent as anxiety or depression, around 1,250,000 people in the UK suffer from an eating disorder according to figures from the charity Beat[39].

The number of people being diagnosed and entering inpatient treatment for eating disorders in England alone has increased at an average of 7%

year on year since 2009[40,41]. This could be due to the pressure of modern life, the trend for aspirational living, or our overexposure to 'perfect' celebrities and the internet, or on a positive note are medical services being able to better satisfy an unmet need?

Either way it is important to bear in mind that one in ten people with an eating disorder will die from their condition, and although 45% of people do make a full recovery, swift treatment is essential, according to Beat. Clients or their parents who spend a long time covering up what is happening would be well advised to act immediately and tell everyone concerned so that a comprehensive treatment approach can be planned.

Anyone can be affected by an eating disorder at any age, and it's not always linked to body image. Disordered eating can be a way of asserting control, and anorexia or bulimia may develop because of stressful life events. Genetics do play a role in some cases, as people with a certain gene are more likely to develop the condition depending on environmental factors [42,43].

In Chapter 10 I discuss the newly termed 'orthorexia' which is supposed to include those who are obsessed with eating healthy foods. I am aware of bias in the media against those who are raising awareness of unhealthy eating habits and promoting healthy eating, but this is not orthorexia or anorexia. Healthy eating is just common sense.

Why is stress so harmful?

Stress seems to be part of our modern age, but what exactly does this overused word mean? Stress may be defined as 'a temporary state of emotional strain or tension, resulting from adverse or demanding circumstances'. The problem in today's world is that stress is almost constant. We're under unrelenting pressure both at home and at work, with research from the mental health charity Mind revealing that one in five of us has taken time off due to stress (www.mind.org.uk).

Of course, we need some stress to motivate us into action; this is why the hormone cortisol, which is often associated with stress, isn't all bad.

If our bodies are working as they should, our cortisol levels will peak in the morning, giving us the big surge of energy we need to get going, and then should begin to drop off later in the day. This is known as the Cortisol Awakening Response (CAR).

The problem is that, for many of us, our cortisol levels remain permanently high. Under prolonged stress, our bodies are endlessly flooded with cortisol, our blood pressure is raised, and our hearts beat faster. In the short term, this physical response might well make us sharper, faster and stronger, but biologically this is only meant to be a short-term fix. Many of us live in a constant state of stress, putting our bodies under intense strain (you can test your cortisol levels, see Chapter 11).

How does stress affect us physically?

Immune system

Stress reaches beyond the heart. During the fight, flight or freeze (FFF) response, the physiological response to an acute, short-term stress stimulus, your immune responses may be temporarily up-regulated. However, chronic, long-term stress, when your stress button is constantly 'on', causes the opposite, with suppression of your immune response, making us less able to detect and fight infections[44]. Indeed, stress has been linked to faster rates of HIV progression and AIDS onset, and an increased frequency of complications for AIDS sufferers[45].

Heart disease

We have already discussed earlier how stress can take its toll on your waistline. Being under stress can affect where fat is deposited. Studies have revealed that people under constant stress are more likely to gain visceral fat around their waist[46], making them more vulnerable to cardiovascular disease and type 2 diabetes. Furthermore, when you are under stress, your blood vessels constrict, raising blood pressure. German researchers reported recently that people who were constantly exposed to loud traffic were more at risk of having a heart attack because of the stress on their bodies[47].

Cancer

An Australian research project on mice found that high stress levels caused cancer to spread faster[48]. There is evidence that stress in humans could affect processes involved in fighting cancer such as DNA repair and cellular ageing[45]. In fact, some oncologists suggest that cancer patients should be offered anxiety-reducing therapy at the beginning of chemotherapy because of the likely interaction between stress and cancer progression.

Skin

Recently, dermatologists have reported a rise in midlife acne, especially amongst women. Stress has been linked to acne and psoriasis onset and/or severity[49,50]. Doctors have even started treating people suffering from skin conditions with mindfulness in a bid to reduce their stress levels. A client of mine who developed terrible acne at 45 undertook the RYG programme and yoga classes and is now acne free.

Psychological problems

Too much stress over long periods not only affects your memory and other cognitive functions, but if left untreated, chronic stress will affect our mental health. Sometimes it isn't clear where stress ends and a more serious problem begins, but if your thoughts, behaviour and feelings are all consistently negative, it could be time to seek out some mental and physical health support at www.maphealthsolutions.com or a local provider of your choice.

What causes stress?

If you become chronically overwhelmed by stress, you are at risk of developing a mental health problem. Here we will talk about some of the most common mental health challenges.

Today, our stress response is more likely to be triggered by emotional strains rather than real physical threats. In an age dominated by social media, we are on show all the time, and the pressure to look good and to adopt a certain lifestyle is more prevalent than ever. Added to this, most of us are working longer hours, often for less money, and we are living in a time when there seems to be little political or economic stability in the world. According to the 2017 Physiological Society report, 'Stress in Modern Britain' [51], aside from the death of a loved one, divorce and redundancy, other top modern stressors involve fear of terrorism, debt, commuting, and even going on holiday.

There are other factors that make people more susceptible to stress, and through my work as a therapist I have observed that adults who experienced childhood abuse are often more vulnerable to its effects. This is because they tend to exhibit several different mostly unconscious behavioural traits such as self-doubt, low self-esteem, defensiveness, indecisiveness and introversion. They are also statistically more likely to self-harm or to develop addictions [52,53].

Loneliness is another major cause of stress. A recent American study involving 3.5 million people showed that being socially isolated doubled the risk of a premature death [54]. This could be due to loneliness activating the fight or flight response, thereby increasing levels of the protein fibrinogen in the blood, which can raise blood pressure and lead to atherosclerosis [55]. This connection was further emphasised at the 2018 European Society of Cardiology's nursing congress where they presented evidence that people who live alone but have an active social circle don't seem to run the same risks of heart disease.

Burnout is a relatively new term, used to describe physical and emotional exhaustion, apathy and loss of motivation. It is both a cause of stress and a consequence of it. Luckily the warning signs creep up slowly, and may include the following symptoms:

- Fatigue and insomnia

- Lack of energy

- Loss of appetite

- Forgetfulness

- Symptoms of anxiety and depression

Before you get to this stage, there are things you can do to keep exhaustion at bay. Try at least one of the strategies below and see what effect it has on your wellbeing:

- Learn to say no and to delegate

- Make a journal to track your stress triggers

- Spend more time on hobbies and fun activities

- Meditate or attend a mindfulness workshop

- Cut back from devices and social media

...and relook at the suggestions listed under Depression above and *Reset Your Gut* to reduce your stress levels.

Summing up

- Talking therapies are effective but they are more powerful when used in conjunction with healthy changes to nutrition and lifestyle

- The brain is sensitive to nutritional input

- Foods high in sugar release dopamine in the brain leading to cravings

- Stress is associated with suppressed immunity, heart disease and cancer

- An unbalanced microbiome and nutritional imbalance are associated with depression

Notes:

Notes:

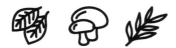

CHAPTER 5

Treatment and therapies for mental health

Nowadays, there are many available therapies and treatments to help us deal with stress and mental health problems that affect so many of us.

Talking therapy or psychotherapy involves discussing and working with mental or emotional challenges to fully understand them and allow you to develop appropriate strategies to help you cope. There are many options: Cognitive Behavioural Therapy (CBT), Counselling Psychology, Psychodynamic Psychotherapy, Emotional Freedom Techniques – Google your options, they are endless. The most important thing is finding a therapist you 'click' with as the therapeutic relationship is essential[12]. I encourage all my clients to follow the *Reset*

Your Gut programme and do appropriate functional tests in conjunction with a talking therapy to get long-lasting results.

Choosing the appropriate talking therapy is a personal choice. While I was training in CBT I was working with a client suffering from 'health anxiety'. I presented the case to a group supervision forum, mostly composed of psychodynamic therapists, and was overwhelmingly advised to investigate further on why the client (who was gay) had not come out yet to his family. They suggested I allowed him to be 'held' in therapy so that he could consider his 'avoidance'.

I reiterated this to the client and he was very clear: "I choose CBT to get strategies to deal with my health anxiety. If I suddenly had a eureka moment after a lot of navel gazing that explained why I had it, then what good is that? I would still not know how to cope with it! And not coming out has nothing to do with my health anxiety, I am just waiting till I finish university, that is my choice."

So, it is horses for courses. Another client needed the 'held treatment' to function, she had to have a session every week. In this case, a psychodynamic approach would be more appropriate.

Therapeutic methods, and indeed therapists themselves, come in many shapes and sizes, so it pays to do your research. If you think you may benefit from therapy, look up any therapists in your local area and the methods they employ and assess what you think will work best for you. Here's a bit of information to get you started.

Talking therapies

Cognitive Behavioural Therapy (CBT)

CBT is a popular therapy that helps you challenge the automatic negative thoughts, beliefs and attitudes that shape your experiences and behaviour. By working with a therapist, you can challenge, and hopefully change, unhelpful or unpleasant patterns of thought. It helps you recognise when negative thoughts and feelings are being translated into unhelpful behaviour. CBT helps people to remember that it is not the difficult child, the demanding boss or friend, or the long commute that is making them feel bad, it's their reactions to them. Whilst you might not be able to change your circumstances, you can certainly reframe how you react, and CBT can be a powerful tool to help you achieve this.

A study carried out recently by researchers at the University of North Carolina and Danube University looked at the efficacy of antidepressants and CBT and found that there was no significant difference between the two strategies in all the studies published between 1990 and 2015[3]. In the UK, the NHS is offering CBT as the first course of treatment for women suffering with PMS (premenstrual syndrome) deemed severe enough to 'affect daily functioning'.

Neuro-Linguistic Programming (NLP)

NLP is a therapeutic technique widely used in the business sector for corporate training and leadership skill development. It is based on the premise that we are often being held back by viewing the world from our own limited perspective rather than seeing the world as it is. By working closely with a therapist, you can learn to work on your communication skills, boost your self-esteem and increase your confidence.

Since its conception in the 1970s, NLP has been used widely by both therapists and life coaches to help people identify and achieve their goals, and to harness opportunities as they arise. It is also used by those looking to break negative habits, overcome trauma and phobias, and gives clients the ability to model effective behaviour. There are many in the scientific community who do not think there is sufficient evidence to empirically 'prove' the efficacy of NLP but, speaking anecdotally, I've observed incredible results in my clients when using NLP to boost their motivation to change their lifestyle habits.

New Code NLP is based on the law of attraction, a concept founded on the idea that we all have the capacity to see our dreams come true and to realise our deepest wishes with the help of visualisation. Therapists use hypnotic language to engage the client's unconscious mind while they are still awake. I also use hypnotherapy as a complementary technique, although not as a primary modality, as the evidence looking at the possible mechanisms for hypnosis are inconclusive[4]. However, I have found it useful in reducing stress in my clients, and a meta-analysis of the therapeutic value of hypnosis concluded: "Hypnosis was superior to controls with respect to the reduction of pain and emotional stress during medical interventions as well as the reduction of irritable bowel symptoms"[5].

Emotional Freedom Technique (EFT)

Also known as Tapping, EFT is a branch of Energy Psychology that has evolved from ancient Chinese medical techniques and thus acts as a bridge between western cultures and traditional eastern medicine. Studies carried out by the EFT community showed that it is particularly effective for treating stress[6]. The technique stimulates the body's meridian points, or 'acupoints' (the key areas where life-energy, referred to as 'qi' or 'chi' flows), by tapping on the area while having the patient focus on specific fears or unresolved trauma. The idea is that a therapist can access the body's energy, helping to bring it back into balance, and thus diminish the power of the negative memory.

It has also been found that the related practice of acupuncture can reduce the stimulation of the amygdala[7], an area of your brain found to be overactive when you are stressed and anxious. Existing EFT trials that fulfil the criteria of the American Psychological Association on Empirically Validated Treatments reported a significant decrease in anxiety levels compared to the control[8]. The study further reports that EFT was "highly effective in reducing depressive symptoms in a variety of populations" [9].

Anecdotally, I have found EFT (and Energy EFT, a modality that looks at all emotions as energy and aims to release or increase the energy created by emotion) incredibly useful in releasing trauma for clients. One client who was repeatedly raped by her father between the ages of four and seven, and who had dealt with this trauma by supressing her memories, experienced her past coming back to haunt her just before she was to get married. The local mental health authority decided she needed to be put in a mental health institution for her own safety.

I saw her on her release, and after she had got married, but she was clearly still very distressed by the memories of the traumatic events in her past. It was clear to me intuitively that she was overusing her fight or flight system, and although her brain had adapted to the heightened adrenalin and cortisol levels to allow her to function, this state was unsustainable for her (I had wanted to test her cortisol levels, but it was not within her budget).

The way EFT purports to heal trauma is to break the stress cycle response so the brain can effectively live in the present without feeling in danger or stressed. When dealing with the fallout from major trauma, as in the case of Post Traumatic Stress Disorder, the prefrontal cortex (an area that allows you to think logically) closes and you are left only with the limbic system that governs emotions. I worked with this client to release the negative energy around her memories, and although she could not forget what happened, recalling the events no longer triggered a stress response.

EFT has been used successfully to alleviate PTSD in combat veterans[10] and practitioners believe that, though it does not fit into typical contemporary medical treatments[11], the methods may be changing some basic assumptions of medicine and psychology. There are also implied cost savings associated with EFT treatment compared to other current approaches. Conditions that had previously been considered intractable, like PTSD, are rapidly remediated. Co-morbid (more than one) conditions, whether psychological such as anxiety and depression, or physiological such as TBI (traumatic brain injury) and pain, improve simultaneously[12]. However, further empirical research is undoubtedly needed to solidify these claims.

When Elizabeth Mason, a psychotherapist, studied the use of energy psychology, she found it was a valuable supplement to an integrative practice[13]. I would agree with this: EFT acknowledges that stress can continue, even though the body is no longer biologically threatened, and it facilitates the release of this stress energy.

Mindfulness is a form of meditation and for some a 'way of being' that focuses our consciousness completely in the moment. By being present, you can learn to observe your thoughts and feelings objectively rather than reacting to them, thus freeing yourself from cycles of negative thought. In a recent study carried out by the BBC programme *Trust Me, I'm A Doctor,* volunteers who used a mindfulness app every day for eight weeks saw an impressive 58% increase in their Cortisol Awakening Response.

Furthermore, research carried out at the University of Oxford revealed that mindfulness-based cognitive therapy (MBCT) stopped almost as many people from sliding back into depression as medication[14]. I explain to my clients that it is very hard to walk forwards whilst looking backwards, ie that we cannot look where we are going if we are thinking about the past.

I personally have suffered from PTSD and, in a perverse way, it has been a gift that has informed my clinical practice. Although I still experience symptoms from time to time, the techniques I have learned through therapy (especially EFT) in conjunction with mindfulness, exercise, sleep, good friends and eating well, has enabled me to let go of fear and move forwards. PTSD UK recommends on its website the use of EFT for sufferers.

Antidepressants

In the last year, more than 70 million prescriptions for antidepressants have been issued in the UK alone. As our dependence on these so-called 'happy pills' increases, there is also increasing debate over their efficacy and possible negative side effects, not to mention the stigma surrounding their use. So, do they really work? Many users insist that medication helped them to regain mental balance, and some claim that antidepressants saved their lives. Indeed, Dr Helen Stokes, chair of the Royal College of General Practitioners (RCGP), claims that antidepressants are very effective for patients with moderate to severe anxiety or depression.

For example, research at the University of Oxford identified 21 antidepressants that were more effective at treating depression than placebos[15]. It is worth remembering that there are many different types of antidepressant medications, each with their own side effect profiles, and not all are equally effective in treating all conditions[16]. If you are considering taking antidepressants, this is something to be discussed in depth with your GP or healthcare provider.

Many users of antidepressants have experienced negative side effects, ranging from increased anxiety, headaches, sexual dysfunction, to weight gain and even fatigue. This does not mean the drugs are ineffective, but does suggest it may be worth considering alternatives to chemical interventions, as explained in the book by Dr Joanna Moncrieff *The Myth of the Chemical Cure*[17] where she proposes that drugs work by creating altered mental states, suppressing the symptoms of psychiatric disorders rather than targeting the underlying causes.

What can you do to avoid taking drugs?

It is my view that mental health and physical health are inextricably linked, which is why I encourage my clients to adopt healthy lifestyle habits (such as following the *Reset Your Gut* programme) in conjunction with talking therapy to promote optimum mental and physical health. I also employ strategies to help them overcome resistance and lack of motivation and adopt changes in basic behaviours, like exercise, sleep, and eating well. As Dr Chatterjee said: "I believe GPs need to learn more about the functional medicine approach, as well as nutritional science, and they need to engage people in behavioural change." Sadly, the relationship between physical health, nutrition, motivation and positive health outcomes is not emphasised enough in the current medical curriculum.

Behavioural changes

Some of these have chapters of their own but are repeated here for clarity.

Eat well – if you are under constant stress it is important to maintain a balanced diet for your essential nutrients (see Chapter 2). For example, B vitamins, found in green vegetables and nuts, not only improve brain function but have also been found to improve your mood as well[18].

It seems you might really be able to eat yourself happy!

Exercise – moving to get your blood pumping is an effective way to tackle depression[19]. In one study, participants were asked to walk quickly on a treadmill for 30 minutes over a ten-day period. At the end, researchers noted a significant reduction in depression markers amongst those taking part[20]. It has been suggested that physical pursuits which require a lot of concentration or coordination have the best effect on your mental health as you simply can't ruminate or dwell on your problems.

Find your passion – research reveals that finding a hobby you love not only reduces stress but it might even prolong your life and reduce your chances of developing dementia[21].

Embrace nature – according to researchers at the University of Illinois[22], being able to see trees (even if you live in a city) significantly reduces stress. This appears to validate the commonly held belief that spending time in the natural world can soothe us and improve our mood. Exercising outdoors may also be more satisfying and lead to greater contentment levels compared with exercising in a gym[23] and, as an extra bonus, it's free!

Read – it might well be a cliché, but it seems that losing yourself in a book really can calm frazzled nerves. According to research carried out at the University of Sussex[24] just six minutes of reading can reduce your stress levels by 68% and is more effective than listening to music (61%) having a cup of tea (54%), or taking a walk (42%). Unfortunately, scanning your smartphone for new texts or scrolling through social media does not have the same beneficial effects – it's far better to escape into a novel. Another study, conducted on children aged between eight and ten, revealed a strong positive correlation between reading abilities, how much the children read, and how much white matter (the part of the brain responsible for carrying nerve impulses to other areas) there was in their brains[25].

Altruism – the drive to help others without any selfish gain. This is an inherent quality in humans, as well as across many other species. A study was carried out to investigate the links between stress altruism and mortality[26]. It turns out that people who were inclined to help others and carry out selfless acts are significantly less affected by personal stress (unless they are in stressful carer situations). Another study involved a large group of older people (mean age around 60) of which 3,500 were caregivers and 24,900 were not[27]. The participants were followed up after six years and a significantly larger proportion of caregivers survived compared to non-caregivers.

These studies highlight the effectiveness of altruism and social interaction in humans: being there when people need you not only helps them, but may help you live a longer, more fulfilling life. Humans are naturally gregarious, as my father once told me… "we need other people as much as they need us."

Positivity – I have always believed that having a positive outlook is good for your health, and now there is proof that being upbeat can prolong your life. A study by researchers in Denmark monitored more than 600 patients with serious heart disease, revealing that those with a 'glass half full' mentality were 58% more likely to live longer than the 'glass half empty' patients, and this may be due to the evidence that those with a positive attitude were twice as likely to take exercise[28].

Overall, positive people not only have better heart health, but they are less prone to infections, have quicker recovery times and generally live longer. Interestingly, they tend to have lower cortisol levels too and are therefore less likely to suffer from stress[29]. So next time you feel like moaning or groaning, it is definitely worth slapping on a smile and focusing on something you feel grateful for. Like anything else, positivity is a skill that becomes easier with practice.

Happy hormones

Everyone is vulnerable to the negative effects of stress, so it is important to remember that we all have the power to feel good too.

Dopamine is a hormone that contributes to controlling the pleasure and reward centres of our brain. Low levels of dopamine can lead to depression and impaired executive function (our ability to plan ahead and get things done). You can boost your dopamine levels by achieving goals, however small – anything from getting the kids to school on time, tidying your desk or getting a promotion. You can also naturally boost your dopamine levels by eating plenty of fresh fruit and vegetables.

Oxytocin is commonly known as the 'love hormone' and is responsible for inducing a feeling of calm and wellbeing in response to physical touch, orgasm and breastfeeding. It is essential for creating strong bonds, and plays a role in strengthening your immune system[30]. Laughter, hugs and receiving and/or giving gifts also boosts oxytocin.

Serotonin is another 'happy hormone' released when you feel important or have a sense of belonging. It plays a role in regulating your mood, sleep, and response to pain, and may also impact on the functioning of the gut. Serotonin levels become diminished if you are lonely or depressed, but can be boosted by reflecting on past successes or practising gratitude. Serotonin production can also be boosted by exposure to sunshine[31].

Endorphins are natural painkillers released by your body in response to stress and may also contribute to alleviating symptoms of anxiety and depression. You can induce endorphin production through exercise and laughter. Eating dark chocolate and spicy food is also believed to help your body release endorphins.

We can live well by encouraging a balance of our 'happy hormones', staying positive, and adopting attitudes and behaviours that are beneficial for our mental and physical health.

Good mental health

We have discussed what happens to you when you are chronically stressed. Your thoughts, feelings and behaviour become consistently negative, sometimes to the extent that you develop anxiety, depression or other psychological problems. But what exactly does good mental health look like?

Psychotherapist Amy Morin, the author of *13 Things Mentally Strong People Don't Do*, has outlined several 'Dos and Don'ts' when it comes to leading a happy and fulfilling life.

The following are behaviours Morin rarely sees in confident, mentally strong people:

- Feeling sorry for themselves

- Playing the victim

- Shying away from change

- Worrying about things they can't control

- Trying to please everyone

- A fear of taking risks

- Dwelling on the past

- Repeating mistakes

- Giving up easily

- A fear of being alone

- Thinking the world owes them a living

- Expecting immediate results

- Comparing themselves to others

On the other hand, the following positive behaviours are typically displayed in mentally strong and naturally resilient people:

- Emotional intelligence

- Knowing when to say no

- Regular exercise

- Surrounding themselves with supportive, non-toxic people

- Fearlessness – not letting fear hold them back

- Good sleeping habits

- The ability to forgive and forget

- The ability to embrace failure

- Relentless positivity

How many of these apply to you?

Summing up

- Talking therapies, antidepressants and mindfulness-based cognitive therapy are all possible treatments for stress and mental health issues

- Behavioural changes (such as diet and exercise changes) can also improve mood and mental state

- Exercise is an effective way to tackle depression

- Embracing nature can improve mood

- Try to boost your 'happy hormone' levels by getting some sunshine, achieving small goals and eating plenty of fruit and vegetables

- Maintain a positive attitude

Notes:

Notes:

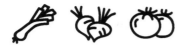

CHAPTER 6

Inflammation

Although most people are probably familiar with the term 'inflammation' – usually used when talking about the redness and swelling around a wound when you cut yourself or sprain something – actually understanding what inflammation is and its potential impact on your health requires some serious explanation.

Inflammation is one of those words often bandied about by medical professionals, but what does it actually *mean*? In the broadest sense, inflammation is simply your body's way of defending itself from infection, injury, bacteria and even – as will be discussed later – certain foods. When your immune system detects the presence of a foreign microorganism or object, it responds by automatically sending protective white blood cells to any part of your body that it believes to be under attack. This process is necessary for the removal of damaged cells, the elimination of toxins and pathogens, and to promote repair after injury or infection.

Inflammation is caused by fluid and white blood cells leaking into the surrounding tissues, causing swelling, and in fact supporting the healing process. As you can see, inflammation is vital to the body's ability to protect itself from immediate danger and damage. However, it's not all good news: chronic, long-term inflammation can cause serious damage, and I mean long term.

Who knows or can prove how long the non-communicable diseases listed below take to develop? Years, decades? What we do know is that they do it with stealth and sometimes with no symptoms until suddenly you have a full-blown health issue. Best avoided!

So, unlike acute inflammation, the short-lived processes occurring after an injury or in response to conditions such as appendicitis, tonsillitis, dermatitis and sinusitis, chronic inflammation is like a fire that burns through your body all the time, and for a long time. It doesn't always cause pain or symptoms (at least not at first) but it has nonetheless been described as a 'silent killer', responsible for damaging cells and ultimately making you far more vulnerable to a whole range of diseases and serious health conditions.

Chronic inflammation can occur over a number of years and can be the precursor to several major non-communicable diseases (NCDs) – conditions not caused by an infectious agent. What do you think cancer[1], diabetes[2], arthritis[3], heart disease, psoriasis, IBS, thyroid malfunction, obesity, autoimmune diseases, some mood disorders[4], cognitive decline and common allergic conditions like asthma and eczema all have in common? That's right – inflammation!

Chronic inflammation has been linked to many environmental and lifestyle factors, meaning that the lifestyle choices you make now may influence your chances of developing NCDs as much as 30 or 40 years down the line. This chapter, and subsequent chapters, will therefore be spent exploring how to avoid risk factors and incorporate healthy lifestyle habits that will decrease your risk of developing chronic inflammatory conditions.

What does inflammation do to your body?

Cancer

In a world where someone is diagnosed with cancer every two minutes (Cancer Research UK statistics), it is becoming more important than ever that we attempt to understand the causes of the disease and what we can do to reduce our chances of getting it. There is growing evidence suggesting that cancer is inextricably linked with chronic inflammation – a condition that causes your body to believe that its own healthy tissues are a threat and therefore need to be destroyed – suggesting that to tackle one it's best to start by tackling the other.

It is clear from research that inflammation plays more of a part in some cancers than in others. Unfortunately, people who suffer from inflammatory bowel disease (IBS) are 70% more likely to develop bowel cancer than people without this condition[5]. Similarly, there is a well-established link between inflammation and mouth cancer: a recent study revealed that post-menopausal women with poor dental hygiene were 14% more likely to develop cancer than those with healthy teeth and gums[6].

Dr Tanya Malpass, author of *Bob the Blob's Blog* (referring to a malignant brain tumour she took to calling 'Bob the Blob'), survived cancer against all odds and has some very pragmatic suggestions to help other people do the same. She says that whatever path you decide to take when it comes to tackling cancer, it's essential to do the research, find what works for you and have faith in a positive outcome. From experience, she also recommends eating in such a way as to reduce inflammation. Kelly Turner, a researcher investigating common themes in long-term cancer survivors, found that all subjects interviewed had made positive changes to their lifestyle and, in addition, had absolute faith that those changes would work.

Unfortunately, the power of hope, expectation, belief and determination can't be tested in a double-blind study. But from where I'm sitting, I think these results really speak for themselves.

The *Reset Your Gut* programme is specifically designed with nutritionists and doctors to reduce the consumption of inflammatory foods.

Arthritis

Some types of arthritis, albeit not all, are the result of misdirected inflammation. This includes rheumatoid arthritis, a condition in which your immune system attacks your body's joints, resulting in inflammation that can harm them even further. Symptoms include pain, stiffness and red, swollen joints. Certain types of arthritis (rheumatoid) and gouty arthritis[7] have also been linked to chronic inflammation, and this is associated with joint damage and loss of mobility over time[8].

Diabetes

Many people with type 2 diabetes test positive for certain molecules typically associated with chronic inflammation (see Chapter 11 for available tests), suggesting inflammation may be contributing to the development of the disease. Doctors suspect that obesity and excess abdominal fat can cause inflammation, and that this may make it harder for your body to use insulin effectively[9]. Other research has shown that inflammation may activate proteins that block insulin production.

Whatever the precise cause, as the rates of diabetes continue to rise, making changes to your diet and lifestyle to protect your body from chronic inflammation seems like a very sensible idea[10].

Dementia

Chronic brain inflammation is often seen in people with dementia, and appears to play a key role in the development of the disease. Researchers based at the University of Oxford found that people admitted to hospital with autoimmune conditions (illnesses caused by the immune system attacking the patient's own body tissues) are more likely to be admitted for dementia later in life[11]. Your brain is very susceptible to inflammation, which can alter the blood flow to the brain and ultimately lead to tissue damage, cognitive decline and the creation of proteins linked to the development of Alzheimer's[12] (see Chapter 12 for more details).

Cutting edge research is now showing inflammation in the brain may, in fact, be linked to what's going on in our gut[13]. This is a massive paradigm shift for the medical community and has raised many questions that we have yet to find answers to. While there is still much we don't know, these discoveries suggest that we can influence our susceptibility to conditions like dementia and Alzheimer's by altering the way we live and eat every day. The more tools we have in our toolbox to help us live better and healthier lives, the greater our chances of maintaining good mental and physical wellbeing, both now and later in life.

It is important that the changes you make are long lasting and not just a diet that you go on for a period of time. The RYG programme is designed to enable people to make lasting lifestyle changes.

Leaky gut syndrome[26]

There is growing evidence that inflammation across the body can stem from the disrupted flora of the intestine.

The gut is lined by epithelium – a one-cell-thick layer – with bacteria and different proteins lying on top to form a mucus layer. The cells of the epithelium associate with each other very tightly but still possess limited permeability: they allow specific substances to pass though the barrier. Normally it's just water and ions, but there is a hypothesis that certain factors can increase and decrease gut permeability; in other words make it easier or harder for substances to pass through, and when they do they trigger an immune reaction in your body that leads to inflammation[14]. Western diets high in trans fats (see Chapter 2) and sugars as well as alcohol can increase permeability.

The barrier they form is associated with lymphoid tissue, which is an integral part of the immune system, and increases in permeability are communicated to the immune system, which in turn steps in with a protective role triggering inflammation.

This increase in permeability is sometimes called leaky gut syndrome and links between inflammation, the microbiome and the affected barrier have been demonstrated in animal models. So where does the microbiome come in? It is thought that some bacteria help reverse the increase in permeability, promoting the functional integrity of the barrier[27]. And, vice versa, pathogenic ('bad') bacteria can compromise it. So it is important to maintain a balanced microbiome, and once again the RYG programme can help to balance your gut bacteria and reduce your inflammatory load.

Other inflammatory conditions

I've mentioned a few of the major conditions associated with chronic inflammation, but there are plenty of other modern illnesses in which inflammation is thought to play a role: asthma, eczema, hay fever, hives, inflammatory bowel disorders[15], MS – the list goes on. Furthermore, repeated exposure to allergens such as dust and pollen is also thought to lead to inflammation that, if left untreated, can cause tissue damage[12]. This is why controlling inflammation might well prove to be one of the most preventative health measures you can take today.

Tests for inflammation

While acute inflammation has some obvious symptoms (eg redness, swelling, pain and heat), chronic inflammation is often significantly harder to spot. Possible symptoms include:

- Fatigue

- Mouth sores

- Chest pain

- Abdominal pain

- Fever

- Rash

- Joint pain

Unfortunately, sufferers may display just a few (or indeed none) of the above symptoms, making some chronic inflammatory conditions difficult to diagnose. This being said, there are a couple of routine blood tests you can request if you're concerned about inflammation. A 'CRP blood test', for instance, measures the amount of C-reactive protein (a substance released by your liver in response to inflammation) in your blood and can be used as a general marker of inflammatory conditions. CRP tests, and related tests, will be discussed in depth in Chapter 11.

Inflammation and your microbiome

Research suggests that inflammation can be caused by major disruptions to the balance of your microbiome. Given the central role of the microbiome in both physical and mental health, this suggests that combating inflammation and rebalancing your microbiome is vital for good health. Sadly, doctors tend to respond to physical problems by providing drugs like ibuprofen, which can disrupt the microbiome even more, and lead to… wait for it… the need for more drugs!

Prescription drugs often treat the symptom, not the cause. It is like a leaking roof approach where you plug the hole with a temporary repair but ultimately it is best to find the cause of the leak. The gut is the same. If it is compromised and allows 'foreign invaders' into the blood stream you will initially feel nauseous or full of air, have a headache, or break out in spots. Over the long term it will stimulate your immune system into an inappropriate inflammation reaction (see earlier in this chapter for a full description of leaky gut).

What can you do to avoid inflammation?

Look at your diet

According to leading cardiologist Dr Aseem Malhotra, a Mediterranean diet complete with plenty of oily fish and fresh fruit and vegetables is the best way to reduce inflammation. This diet is high in plant-based compounds such as polyphenols and good fats like omega-3 fatty acids that act as anti-inflammatories. This being said, while dietary fatty acids can contain anti-inflammatory chemicals that your body can't make by itself[16], a diet high in saturated fats is thought to reduce the production of these highly beneficial agents. Dr Aseem Malhotra (in line with what I suggested in Chapter 2) suggests eating animal fats in moderation and focus instead on consuming the good fats found in products such as nuts and olive oil. (The RYG programme has vegan and vegetarian options which are designed to fulfil all nutrient requirements.)

Malhotra also supports the increasingly common view that excess sugar consumption is a risk factor in many chronic conditions. In fact, in his article 'The Truth about Fat and Sugar' he goes as far as saying that sugar consumption has an impact on heart health due to its inflammatory properties[17]. Similarly, after a two-year review involving 16 scientists, the Swedish Council on Health Technology concluded that a diet incorporating plenty of good fats and limiting carbohydrates is both best for weight loss and for reducing several markers of inflammation and cardiovascular risk in the obese. In short, as Dr Eenfeldt told their conference: "You don't get fat from eating fatty foods, just as you don't turn green from eating green vegetables."

Fibre: The indigestible part of plants, is also essential to any anti-inflammatory diet as high-fibre foods such as fruit and vegetables contain compounds called phytonutrients that have anti-inflammatory properties[18] and of course feed your all-important bacteria in your microbiome.

Low GI: As we discussed in Chapter 2, sticking to foods with a low glycaemic index (GI) is a great way of reducing your glycaemic load (GL) and regulating your blood sugar levels. Not only is this a good idea to reduce your chances of developing cancer (vast quantities of sugar and carbohydrates feed cancer cells), but there is also evidence to suggest that people who eat a diet rich in slowly digested carbohydrates like legumes and lentils, as well as high-fibre fruit and vegetables, have significantly lower levels of the inflammation marker C-reactive protein[19].

Herbs and spices: Current research is looking into the possible beneficial effects of turmeric[22] in treating arthritis, Alzheimer's disease and some other inflammatory conditions like cancer. However, this research is a good example of the distortion of research by the press and something suddenly becomes a superfood. It has been reported in many tabloid articles that eating more curry containing turmeric helps protect against cancer. This is partly true: curcumin, a chemical in turmeric, has been shown to have anti-proliferative effects in many cancers[23].

However, as curcumin is poorly absorbed into the blood, a few grams of the chemical is needed for there to be detectable levels in the blood, and you would need to eat around 100g of turmeric to get a few grams of curcumin – this would require impossibly excessive curry eating! Research is ongoing about improving curcumin bioavailability and anticancer potential for therapy[24], in the meantime eating it will do no harm.

Ginger: Has been used for hundreds of years to treat constipation, colic and other gastrointestinal problems as well as rheumatoid arthritis pain[25]. Why not throw some in your stir-fry or a curry next time you're in the kitchen? Healthy and delicious.

Good digestion

If you want to avoid inflammation, it is essential that you do your best to eliminate any digestive problems and enable your body to absorb the nutrients from your diet efficiently. As you have already discovered in this book, an imbalance in the microbiome of your gut can lead to inflammation in other parts of your body[26]. Allergies and intolerances to certain foods can also cause an inflammatory response, so we recommend getting yourself checked using some of the tests discussed in Chapter 11. If you don't want to go down the testing route, it's possible to tackle problem foods simply by listening to your body; if a certain food seems to put your body under stress, don't eat it!

As you can see, if you want to avoid inflammation it definitely pays to eat well. To get you started, I've included a list of some of the best (and worst) foods you can eat to tackle inflammation.

Anti-inflammatory foods (all included in the RYG programme)

- Fatty cold-water fish (see Chapter 8 for which ones)

- Berries

- Tree nuts (walnuts, almonds, hazelnuts)

- Seeds (flax, linseed, sunflower, pumpkin)

- Mushrooms and other fungi

- Peppers (bell peppers, chillies)

- Garlic

- Olive oil

- Cacao and dark chocolate

- Tomatoes

Foods to avoid

- Sugar

- Alcohol

- Fried food

- Refined flour (pizza, white bread, pasta)

- Dairy

- Artificial sweeteners

- Trans fats

- Processed meats (ham, bacon, sausages)

Reduce stress

So, you've fixed up your diet – what else can you do? Unsurprisingly, stress has also been found to play a role in inflammation, with research showing that chronic stress supposedly suppresses the body's ability to regulate inflammatory responses[27].

Common sources of stress include:

- Physical injury

- Emotional upset

- Infection

- Nicotine

- Environmental toxins

Sustained stress increases levels of the stress hormone cortisol. When the body is overstimulated by cortisol, it gradually adapts and reduces its response to further stimulation. Cortisol has an important anti-inflammatory role, and thus a loss of sensitivity to cortisol reduces inflammation regulation and may lead to the inflammation-associated conditions discussed earlier in the chapter. Cortisol's anti-inflammatory properties are thought to be due to its ability to suppress the production of pro-inflammatory cytokines[28]. Increased inflammation, due to poor lifestyle and diet, leads to elevated levels of cortisol and a weakening of the immune system. This sets the scene for infection and degenerative diseases.

Interesting new studies are looking at the stimulation of the vagus nerve, which is part of a circuit that links the neck, lungs, heart and abdomen to the brain. These studies show how it is possible to directly impact the inflammatory reflex of the vagus nerve which produces the cytokines that cause inflammation. Paul-Peter Tak, the principal investigator of these studies, states: "This approach might be relevant for other inflammatory diseases as well" and could be an alternative to fighting inflammatory conditions with relatively expensive drugs[29].

Stress and heart health

The association between stress, stroke and heart attack has been well known for a while, but it is only relatively recently that scientists are truly starting to understand the link. A study from Harvard Medical School has found that if you are more prone to feel stressed you have heightened activity in your amygdala. This makes you more vulnerable to heart disease as this part of the brain is responsible for telling the body to temporarily produce more white cells, leading to inflammation and the development of plaques on the arteries[30]. This study highlights the importance of reducing your stress levels. Talking therapies and the RYG programme can assist this process working together to promote a happier mind and healthier body.

Learn to relax

It is vital to lower your stress levels if you want to protect your body from the effects of chronic inflammation. Earlier in this book, we looked at different ways to relax including mindfulness, fulfilling hobbies and pastimes, exercise and even talking therapies. If you feel your life is too stressful, perhaps start looking into strategies such as these to help reduce the pressure.

Sleep well

Poor sleep has been shown to cause increased inflammation in your body, and ultimately, a heightened risk of heart disease and stroke. Research undertaken at the University Medical School in Atlanta revealed that those people who consistently get less than six hours' sleep showed elevated levels of three proteins associated with inflammation compared to those who regularly slept between seven and eight hours a night[31].

Keep regular hours

It appears that *when* you sleep might be just as important as *how much* shut-eye you are getting. A study conducted by the World Health Organisation revealed that regular changes to sleep patterns can have a negative impact on your health as it interferes with your circadian rhythms. This not only results in inflammation but may also cause problems with fat and sugar metabolism, making you more vulnerable to cancer and heart disease[32]. So, if you are a shift worker or regularly move between different time zones, it is even more important to make sure you are protecting your body from inflammation in every way possible (see Chapter 10 for more detail on sleep).

Get moving

If you want to increase your chances of enjoying continued good health and reduce your chances of developing arthritis, diabetes or dementia, it's time to get active. Exercise has powerful anti-inflammatory powers. According to a recent American study, just 20 to 30 minutes of moderate exercise a day can make a real difference to our health. This is because it sets off a beneficial chain reaction: your brain and your sympathetic nervous system are both accelerated whilst releasing proteins that help to regulate inflammation[33].

Control your weight

For many years obesity has been associated with increased inflammation. Research has shown that lowering your body mass index (BMI), can also bring your white cell blood count back into the normal range, making you far less vulnerable to the illnesses and health conditions we have already mentioned in this chapter[34].

Get in balance

Ironically, overdoing it at the gym or exercising too much can also increase inflammation in the body and I don't just mean sore muscles. Recent research published in Australia has found that going 'too hard' during training puts the body under strain and can exacerbate conditions such as leaky gut syndrome, which could flood the bloodstream with germs and toxins. Furthermore, excessive exercise puts the body into an almost permanent fight or flight mode, resulting in very high levels of cortisol being released to tackle what the body believes to be inflammation. This can seriously compromise your immune system[35].

Summing up

Chronic long-term inflammation can occur over a number of years and be the precursor to several non-communicable diseases.

- Get at least seven hours' sleep

- Exercise regularly

- Get tested

- Reduce junk food

- Increase fibre and fruit and vegetable intake

- Eat healthy fats

- Try to reduce your stress levels with talking therapies, hobbies or exercise

- Commit to an anti-inflammatory programme such as the *Reset Your Gut* programme

- Maintain a healthy BMI

Notes:

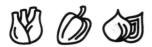

CHAPTER 7

Drugs

The current paradigm in conventional medicine is to treat the inflammatory conditions described in the last chapter and many other conditions with drugs. Certainly, this approach has reduced the discomfort of symptoms for millions of people, but as you read on you will learn that some doctors are looking to get back the balance so that they do no harm, and look at alternatives to drugs whenever possible. I have included drugs in this book because, like the following two chapters about toxins, any unnatural substance has the potential to upset your gut bacteria. So if you have to take drugs it is essential to eat healthily, exercise and reduce your stress.

Prescription drugs

We all know that medication is supposed to keep us healthy, but how much is too much? Shockingly, a recent study by the Cambridge Institute of Public Research revealed that 49% of people over the age of 65 are now taking five different prescription drugs, every day, compared to just

12% in 1997[1]. So, what is going on here? Do all these extra prescriptions represent a huge advance in medical science, or are we simply being persuaded to take medicine we don't need?

In the UK, the number of prescriptions has doubled over the last decade. Many GPs and medics fear that people are now being over medicated, often with negative results[2]. Hospital emergency unit doctors have been shocked by how much they have underestimated the number of opioid (pain killing) prescriptions they actually write out[3].

Polypharmacy (taking multiple prescriptions) can cause all sorts of unwelcome side effects. According to one expert, nearly half of older adults (over 65) "take one or more medications that are not medically necessary"[4]. In addition, some prescription drugs can be highly addictive. Rehab provider UK Addiction Treatment Centres revealed that admissions for people addicted to prescription drugs had increased by 22% between 2015 and 2017[5]. It is a well-known fact that drug companies spend more on PR than on research and development[6].

Terrifying though this is, I am greatly encouraged by the recent growth in the field of functional medicine. At a conference I attended run by the Institute for Functional Medicine, the functional medicine practitioners I spoke to were increasingly dissatisfied with dolling out pills and wanted patients to begin taking a functional route to improve their health through changes to their lifestyle. This approach makes conventional doctors nervous as they've learned to be wary of unproven treatments, but when it comes to improving the health of the nation, I'm of the opinion that it's more important to find out what works!

The RYG programme is used by doctors to educate and motivate their patients to improve what they are putting in their mouths. This debate is a massive one for our society, but surely what matters is that you feel better and the Hippocratic Oath of 'do no harm' is upheld.

In April 2018, the global investment bank Goldman Sachs published a paper titled 'Is curing people a sustainable business model?'. They were investigating gene therapy, a gene editing technique which has the potential to deliver a 'one-shot cure' to hereditary diseases using genetically engineered cells. They concluded that "while this proposition carries tremendous value for patients and society, it could represent a challenge for genome medicine developers looking for sustained cash flow" [7]. Drug companies are driven by bottom line profits and it remains to be seen how they would deal with this loss of cash flow; ultimately their responsibility is to shareholders, not patients.

This discussion is too long to be fully addressed in this book, but there is overwhelming evidence that the pharmaceutical industry, and the medical field in general, has become inextricably entangled with commercial interests leading to a drug-based treatment approach rather than preventative measures [8]. This, in combination with limited nutritional education received by doctors over the course of their degrees, and doctors having very limited appointment times, is dangerous. Addiction to opioid painkillers is being fuelled by a $9m budget that drug companies are spending on inducements for physicians. It has been shown that there is an association between doctors being paid by pharmaceutical companies and the amount of opioids they prescribe [9].

In 2016, 27,000 Americans died from conditions associated with opioid painkiller addiction and many more are dependent on the drugs. As researcher Scott Hadland said: "The pharmaceutical industry must look beyond its bottom line and make changes to its marketing strategies in order to play a role in helping curb opioid overdose deaths" [2].

Encouragingly, medical students from Liverpool University are campaigning for their degrees to include more teaching on nutrition [10]. Furthermore, functional medicine practitioners like Dr Aseem Malhotra and Dr Ranjan Chatterjee have begun writing to the General Medical Council in the UK and the Health Secretary calling for all medical students and practising doctors to be adequately trained in nutrition and lifestyle interventions. Even the editor-in-chief of the *British Medical Journal*, Dr Fiona Godlee, is getting involved, saying: "It's time we recognised that food and nutrition are core to health. There is a growing body of research out there that needs to be published and we want to contribute to that effort."

Doctors are an essential part of delivering the products of drug companies and medics have come to value the industry's input into their jobs, leading to both patient and societal harm[11]. Personally, I believe the best way to deal with this complicated situation is for us to change our lifestyles and reduce our reliance on doctors and prescription drugs.

If your interest is piqued by the role of 'Big Pharma' in modern healthcare, I would recommend watching David Healy's *Time to abandon evidence based medicine?* He suggests that medicine needs to respond and regroup as its credibility is being increasingly challenged. We cannot continue having such a heavy reliance on drugs – both from a social and economic standpoint – and doctors are ideally positioned to become the front line in educating their patients about lifestyle changes they can make to stop this toxic trend.

Antidepressants

As I mentioned earlier in this book, antidepressants are being prescribed at higher levels than ever before. A recent study from the University of Oxford demonstrated the effectiveness of 21 antidepressants in adults with depression[12]. But as the ensuing arguments by experts in their fields showed, it is never that straightforward, as there are a multitude of other approaches for alleviating depression (see Chapter 5). I am personally part of the growing discipline of functional mental health practitioners[13] that focuses on the use of food, limited supplements and functional tests to provide an alternative treatment for mental health disorders, hopefully without a drug prescription. You can read more about it on my website: www.maphealthsolutions.com.

We know what good food does for our mental and physical health, but what exactly do 'happy pills' do to our bodies? There is a need to study the long-term risks associated with prolonged antidepressant treatment[14]. This lack of long-term studies looking at the effects of taking antidepressants for a prolonged period of time isn't meant to scare you. Antidepressants can be a lifeline for people with severe anxiety or depression, but if you want to manage your depression without drugs, or if you're feeling blue and life has thrown out a few curveballs lately, it might be worth asking yourself if therapy or changes to your lifestyle might be worth considering first. However, always talk to your doctor before reducing your drug dose.

Antibiotics

These 'wonder drugs' are currently the best weapons you have for fighting off bacterial infections. However, it's important to remember that antibiotics are completely ineffective against common viral infections like colds and flu. Furthermore, if they're not prescribed properly they can do you more harm than good.

Over-prescription of antibiotics is a serious global health risk as it encourages antibiotic resistance – the growth of bacterial strains that resist treatment. It is essential that antibiotics are taken as per medical advice and only when absolutely necessary[15]. As we have already seen, the use of antibiotics has been shown to have a hugely detrimental effect on your gut – reducing the richness and diversity of your microbiome and potentially inducing widespread effects for both your mental and physical health[16,17]. In some cases the relative levels of beneficial bacteria was not seen, even after one year[18]. However, you should keep in mind that there are many antibiotics, each with a variable potency. So, while some antibiotics may cause long-lasting shifts in the microbiome, this may only be attributed to certain compounds.

You can also take comfort in knowing that after a course of antibiotics, eating foods that are good for your gut can really help you on the road to restoring your gut population. Prebiotics in their purified form (supplements) can increase the relative levels of beneficial bacteria in as little as six weeks[19]. Your gut is extremely sensitive to the foods you eat, so if you want a healthy and balanced gut in the long term, the emphasis should be on lifestyle rather than relying on one-hit changes. The RYG programme can help you rebalance your gut after a course of antibiotics.

Ironically, antibiotics – medication used to combat infection – can actually weaken your body's natural defences. A research study on mice, carried out at the University of Virginia's School of Medicine, revealed that antibiotics had a negative effect on the ability of neutrophils (white blood cells) to travel to the site of the infection, resulting in a suppressed immune response[20]. It's easy to see why researchers and healthcare professionals are continuing to stress that you should only take antibiotics if absolutely necessary.

Methylphenidate

Better known under its many trade names, including Ritalin and Concerta, this stimulant is used to treat attention deficit hyperactivity disorder (ADHD) and narcolepsy. It works by increasing the sensitivity of neurons in your prefrontal cortex[21] and this can help with executive functions like planning, focus, problem solving and organising.

According to the NHS, prescriptions of methylphenidate have doubled in the UK in the last ten years. The evidence suggests it is highly effective for managing ADHD, with 70% of adults and 80% of children seeing a marked improvement in their symptoms by using these stimulants[22]. However, short-term side effects can include a loss of appetite, headaches, insomnia and increased anxiety. In the US, calls to poison centres arising from misuse of these drugs are on the rise, with deliberate abuse accounting for 50% of the cases, while medication errors, including overdose and taking the drugs too frequently, were responsible for most of the cases in children up to 12 years old. Researchers report that this was a 61% rise, which is in line with the rise in ADHA prescriptions[23].

This stimulant doesn't just raise your blood pressure and heart rate, but can cause agitation, irritability, drowsiness, lethargy and vomiting; it can also cause significant weight loss, tics, stunted growth and severe sleeping problems[24]. There is no research yet on the drug's effect on the microbiome, but with side effects like these, I would guess that the bacteria in your gut must be impacted. It is also important to remember that as an amphetamine (like cocaine), this drug can easily be abused and become addictive.

When counselling university students, I found that this drug was being used to help students revise for exams. Sadly, in my work I saw the other side of taking these supposedly 'performance enhancing drugs': increased anxiety, depression and sleep deprivation.

Self-medication

We can all do with a kick-start now and again.

A stimulant is a substance that raises the level of physiological or nervous activity in the body and temporarily increases alertness, mood and awareness by affecting the way the brain works. It produces a stimulating effect on the central nervous system, which in turn can cause a feeling of pleasure, an increase in energy and heightened awareness. Think of that 'buzz' you get when you have your first cup of coffee in the morning. That's your brain reacting to the stimulant in your drink, in this case caffeine. Some stimulants are legal and widely used, and others are addictive and illicit, and as I am sure you know, they all affect your body in different, sometimes catastrophic ways.

Caffeine

Like many people, you may enjoy a daily latte or a few shots of espresso to get you going in the morning. Coffee, like chocolate, is one of those little treats that a lot of us aren't keen to give up. So the question is: do you really need to? To answer this, let's look at the science.

Health benefits

Coffee contains many different compounds, meaning its effects on the body are hard to understand. There are many papers showing beneficial effects, yet more demonise it for negative effects. Caffeine and coffee are not synonymous. So, some of the effects of caffeine could of course be excluded by drinking decaffeinated coffee.

A recent Spanish study involving 451,743 men and women from across Europe concluded that people with higher levels of coffee drinking (over six cups a day) had a lower risk of death by all causes, particularly related to circulatory and digestive disease[25], and four cups of coffee in another study were shown to help our mitochondria, our cells' batteries, to function at an optimum level and promote endothelial cells which help protect the heart[26].

However, before you reach for the cafetière, it's important to note that the researchers could prove no causal link between coffee consumption and their findings, although they did suggest that the polyphenols (plant-derived antioxidants) in coffee might offer some protection to the body[27]. Other recent studies have claimed that higher caffeine intake is associated with a reduced risk of developing Parkinson's disease[28] and dementia as coffee acts on the Nrf2 pathway and helps to amplify the detoxification genes to lower inflammation[29]. It has also been suggested that the polyphenols in coffee can lower the risk of metabolic syndrome[30]. But chronic coffee consumption also seems to alter the gut microbiome, mediating some of the beneficial effects[31].

There is an ongoing debate on whether coffee can increase your metabolic rate[32] both during and after exercise if taken before your workout. But, as always, there are two schools of thought, with some studies showing that consuming coffee one hour prior to exercise can improve endurance performance, and others stating that the body can be immune to the effects of the caffeine[33]. I think we should try to consume everything in moderation as chronic coffee consumption can alter the microbiome[31].

In 2018, a judge in California ruled that coffee shops like Starbucks must start putting up warning notices that their drinks may cause cancer. However, the science behind this claim is a little murky. Although coffee *does* contain acrylamide – which becomes carcinogenic when heated to very high temperatures – this is unlikely to affect your cancer risk as even your extra-extra hot cappuccino never gets *that* hot! Furthermore, the University of Milan has published evidence that coffee may confer some protection against endometrial cancer[34], while a UK-based study has found a decreased risk of liver cancer among coffee drinkers[35]. This suggests that coffee might, in fact, help in the fight against cancer.

Is it addictive?

Clearly coffee has some fantastic health benefits, but (and isn't there always a 'but'?) excess caffeine can leave you feeling irritable, anxious and it may well interfere with your sleep. It is important to remember that, however socially acceptable it might be, caffeine is still technically a 'drug' and it is very easy to become psychologically and physically dependent on it. Just drinking one large cup of coffee a day could leave you reliant on its effects – if you miss your daily 'dose', you'll know about it.

Symptoms of caffeine withdrawal include headaches, drowsiness and loss of concentration that, ironically, will probably have you reaching for another coffee just to feel normal. And so the vicious cycle continues. Also, coffee can affect you in different ways, depending on what you have eaten beforehand, as it can increase your metabolism and make you feel hungry depending on what you have eaten. If you have had a high-carb, low-fat and low-protein breakfast, a coffee mid-morning will most likely have you reaching for a snack.

Alternatives

If you are keen to get off the 'buzz-to-slump' caffeine merry-go-round, perhaps it's important to ask yourself why you crave the stuff so much. If it's simply the taste of coffee that you love, then maybe just replace your normal cup with a decaffeinated variety. Alternatively, if your coffee drinking is simply a habit or a much-needed break in a busy day, you could try drinking herbal tea or hot water infused with lemon instead, or even whizz up a fruit/veggie smoothie. For many people, caffeine provides a burst of energy which is addictive in itself. If this sounds like you, it might be worth considering changes to your diet and sleep habits so that you no longer need to rely on stimulants to get you through the day. Consider doing the RYG programme: people who have done so feel energised, sleep much better and have found they no longer crave coffee.

Nicotine

Smoking

There's a well-known saying that 'people smoke for the nicotine but die from the tar'[36]. There's probably no need to remind you of how toxic tobacco is to the body with over 79,000 deaths in England in 2015 alone[37] being caused by tobacco smoking – about ten times the amount caused by alcohol[38].

Highly addictive

Nicotine is highly addictive, giving it a hold on your body that makes it easy to push all reason aside and continue smoking even when you know it's bad for you. It is also particularly potent when delivered through cigarette smoke, as inhalation allows it to enter your bloodstream very quickly (research also suggests that nicotine may not be the only addictive component of smoking[39,40]).

So, what is it about nicotine that is so hard to live without? Nicotine's addictive quality arises from the release of dopamine it triggers, leaving the smoker feeling both stimulated and relaxed. Symptoms of nicotine withdrawal include anxiety, irritability, restlessness, sleep disturbances and weight gain. This perhaps explains why it is so hard to give up cigarettes, with research showing that most quitting attempts fail and relapse back to smoking is common[41].

The good news is that giving up does dramatically reduce your chances of lung cancer, even within five years of quitting. This being said, your risk of cancer is still higher than those who have never smoked[42], suggesting that it's best if you never pick it up in the first place.

Vaping

Electronic cigarettes have gained traction as a safer alternative to smoking tobacco[43] but we currently know very little about the long-term consequences of vaping, and new case reports are now coming through of heavy metals potentially being left behind in the body after vaping[44]. The effect of using electronic cigarettes on the diversity of your gut bacteria may not be as much as tobacco. However, this is still a very new area of research, and validation in larger studies as well as greater understanding of the short- and long-term impact of electronic cigarette use on microbiota composition and function is needed[45].

Alcohol

Although technically classed as a depressant, alcohol can act as a stimulant in small to moderate doses. If a person consumes more than their body can handle, however, they will experience alcohol's classic depressant effects due to its inhibitory effects on the nervous system. A drink or two can give you a buzz, making you feel more sociable, chatty and confident, but sometimes, especially in social situations, it can be difficult to know when to stop.

The more you drink, the greater the effect on your motor functions and higher cognitive functions such as thinking, understanding and reasoning. This results in slurred speech, hazy thinking, slower reaction times, weakened muscles and mobility issues. Alcohol (pure) is used to kill bacteria when nurses use swabs to clean your skin before injection (yes, kill bacteria), so clearly alcohol in beverages will without a doubt disrupt your microbiome if consumed in large quantities.

Safe drinking

When it comes to drinking responsibly, government recommendations suggest that both men and women should stick to a maximum of 14 units of alcohol a week[46]. This is the equivalent of a bottle and a half of wine or five pints of lager. Unsurprisingly, many people are drinking considerably more than this and, as a result, putting themselves at increased risk of heart disease, liver disease, some cancers, and damage to the nervous system[47]. Studies are also showing that thresholds for safe alcohol consumption might need lowering[48,49]. The good news is that the bacteria in your microbiome can be helped back into balance by following the RYG programme if you have had a particularly heavy drinking regime for a few weeks!

Regaining control

If you fear you might be drinking too much, or you find yourself craving a drink in certain situations or at a specific time of day, it's worth stepping back and really thinking about what is driving you to reach for the bottle. Is that extra glass of vino simply a reward at the end of a long day? Do you feel that booze gives you a much-needed confidence boost in certain challenging situations? Or are you using it to block out a problem like a stressful job or a difficult relationship? Excessive drinking is often a multifaceted problem with physical, emotional, social and mental factors all playing a part. If your drinking is excessive it is a good idea to work with a therapist to try to understand what is pushing you towards alcohol as a first step towards breaking this pattern.

Is it all bad?

In 2013 and 2016 studies were done showing that alcohol may have some benefits, with evidence suggesting a daily glass of wine can actually reduce your risk of dementia quite considerably[50]. This is possibly due to the anti-inflammatory and antioxidant properties of the polyphenols found in wine. It has also been suggested that moderate drinking (especially red wine) may well help to protect your heart, another property linked to its polyphenols content[51].

However, a study published in 2017 by *The Lancet* looking at the effect of alcohol consumption on brain structure and function over a 30-year period in 550 people questioned the methodology of earlier studies. In this study, changes in participants' grey and white matter, including hippocampal atrophy, were measured via MRI scans. Cognitive performance was also monitored. The study concluded that alcohol consumption, even at moderate levels, is associated with adverse brain outcomes, and there was no evidence that small amounts of alcohol had a protective effect greater than abstinence[52].

A study in Finland also showed that adolescents who drank heavily showed changes in their metabolites, which was associated with reduced grey matter volume. So, in my view, small amounts of good wine as part of a balanced lifestyle is unlikely to be detrimental!

Illegal and recreational drugs

In 2017, 7,545 hospital admissions in the UK listed drug-related mental health and behavioural disorders as the primary cause, while 14,053 were attributed to poisoning by illicit drugs[53]. So it's easy to see that regular use of illicit substances can have disastrous consequences for your health. Regular use of cocaine, for instance, has been linked to a significantly increased risk of mortality from cardiovascular disease[54,55,56]. This is thought be due to its tendency to increase blood pressure, constrict blood vessels and induce aortic stiffening.

Similarly, MDMA[57] – the party drug that floods your brain with serotonin and generates intense feelings of energy, love and confidence – has been linked to several negative side effects, from minor problems such as dehydration, fatigue and low mood to more serious issues including cardiac arrhythmias and long-term psychiatric problems[58,59,60].

Illegal drugs also tend to be highly addictive, making these possible health consequences more problematic as people keeping coming back for more. It's impossible to predict how your body will react to these drugs until you've taken them, not to mention hard to verify their quality due to their lack of regulation, so it's essential that you exercise caution and think twice before popping that pill.

However, evidence has begun to emerge suggesting that some illegal drugs may prove useful in the management or treatment of certain physical and/or mental disorders. For instance, one of the key components of cannabis – cannabidiol or 'CBD' – has aroused attention in the medical community due to its pain-relieving properties. One study found that lower doses of opioid medications were required to treat patients with chronic pain following the inhalation of vaporised cannabis, with a significant decline in reported levels of pain[61,62].

Cannabis has also been found to improve the symptoms of other illnesses, including childhood epilepsy[63] and Crohn's disease. Psychedelics such as LSD and psilocybin (the active ingredient in magic mushrooms) are also paving the way for a new approach to treating psychological disorders such as anxiety, depression and PTSD by harnessing the tendency of these compounds to induce a more open and malleable state of mind[64].

While this research is still very much in its infancy, and often meets with resistance due to modern society's traditionally negative view of drug use, it holds the potential to revolutionise our approach to disease management. A number of studies reported a link between high levels of cannabis use and an increased risk for the development of psychosis[65, 66]. Although it is not known if cannabis directly causes mental illness, the evidence is abundant enough for researchers in *The Lancet* to warn that "using cannabis could increase [...] risk of developing a psychotic illness later in life"[67].

There is also significant evidence to suggest that people who start using cannabis regularly at a young age increase their risk of developing schizophrenia[68] and depression[69]. As this book is all about having a healthier body and a happier mind today and tomorrow, I wanted to mention both the potential negative long-term effects of recreational cannabis as well as the emerging research in certain diseases.

My advice is to be sensible: do your research and make sure you've fully considered any potential consequences on your wellbeing before giving something a go. While curiosity and experimentation are natural parts of life, it's important to make rational, informed choices, as regular drug use and drug addiction can be very damaging for your health, relationships, finances and ability to continue leading a productive, fulfilling life, and of course the composition of that all-important gut bacteria, as drug taking and healthy eating are not natural bed partners!

Summing up

- You don't need a pill for every ill

- Just because it's legal and popular doesn't mean it's good for you

- Stimulants can be highly addictive and lead to significant side effects

- Enjoy caffeine in moderation

- Instead of self-medicating, try to understand and address the root cause

- RYG programme to boost your energy and avoid kick-starts

Notes:

Notes:

CHAPTER 8

Toxins we consume

In the previous chapters I have outlined the benefits of being active and eating well, but one of the easiest things you can do for your body to reduce inflammation is to make a few small changes and reduce your exposure to the many environmental toxins that go hand in hand with modern living. Again, your gut and microbiome will thank you.

The world is full of toxins, a broad term for those harmful elements in the environment that may damage your body. Technically, a toxin is a pathogen acting inside your body, but I think you will excuse me for using the term as I couldn't think of a more appropriate description. Whilst you can't eliminate them completely, by making a few small changes and by understanding where you come across them in everyday life, you can at least reduce your exposure to them.

I apologise in advance for the technical nature of this chapter, but we live in a technical world. One thing's for sure: if you can wrap your head around the next few pages and manage to avoid some of the toxins I'm about to discuss, you will be doing your mental and physical health a favour, as well as your gut bacteria.

We are what we eat: the importance of reading the label

Did you know the additives in your food and drink are given an E number by the European Food Safety Authority (EFSA) if they are deemed safe for human consumption? If you find this reassuring then move to the next section, but personally, I'm not sure if I trust what they define as 'safe'. At least, I have found some studies that would certainly beg to differ, although the concentrations cited in the studies below are often much higher than those found in packaged foods.

So, what exactly would I look for when checking a food label?

- **E211 sodium benzoate** – commonly used as a preservative, this additive has been linked to triggering hyperactivity and asthma in children[1, 2].

- **E320 butylated hydroxyanisole (BHA)** – found in some cereals, crisps and chewing gum. Research has shown a link to cancer in rats[3]. Human studies have shown that consumption of BHA poses no additional cancer risk[4,5], so the jury is still very much out. My vote? Probably best avoided.

- **E407 carrageenan** – derived from red seaweed and used as a thickener in processed food, it has been linked to ulcers and gastrointestinal cancer in animals[6].

- **E951 aspartame** – this additive is 200 times sweeter than sugar. It is found in processed food and many diet soft drinks and its effect on human cancer risk has been researched for years both by the US National Cancer Institute and European Food Safety

Authority[78]. The evidence for a carcinogenic effect in humans and animal models remains inconclusive [9,10]. Again, the jury is out, but even if you are reassured by a lack of evidence that it is not harmful, you may need to consider its proven effect on appetite (see Chapter 10).

- **E220 sulphur dioxide** – found in fizzy and alcoholic drinks and dried fruit, this additive can bring on asthma attacks in sensitive asthmatic individuals[2].

- **Trans fats** – as mentioned in Chapter 2, trans fats have been linked to high cholesterol, stroke and heart disease[11]. These fats are found naturally in small amounts, but are produced during the industrial hydrogenation process, so avoid food with labels that mention hydrogenated fat in any form.

It is self-evident that most of the food industry is driven by bottom line profits and shows little consideration for your health or their effect on the environment. It is shocking to be told that, since 1997, every single member of government agencies in the USA involved in determining if a particular food additive was safe had financial ties to the industry (either as employees or consultants)[12,13]. The retail food and beverage industry is massive – around 4.7 trillion Euros[14] – and rising worldwide. The flavouring part of this industry is clothed in secrecy as they are choosing to create addictive tasting food, from ingredients that are synthesised in a laboratory, to make people buy more[15]. They literally set out with the intention of hijacking your taste buds to create more sales and profits!

Of course, you always have a choice when it comes to taking control of what you eat. However, as you do not generally have access to the detailed information about the extent or dangers of the additives in your food, it's not always easy to know what the 'right' decision is. Incredibly, USA food manufacturers produce food with different amounts of additives in order to meet the stricter standards of the European Union, meaning they are knowingly serving other countries 'safer' food[12].

Independent scientists commissioned by the European Parliament reviewed the existing science on organic food and concluded it is more environmentally sustainable and contains fewer pesticide residues than non-organic food. One of the most striking points in this report was that they found organic food can help protect children from the brain-altering effects of some neurotoxic pesticides. Similarly, breastfeeding mothers are advised to avoid food sprayed with pesticides as they have been linked to disrupted brain and cognitive development in foetuses[16].

This will hopefully inspire you to stop playing a passive part in this 'chemical warfare' (see section below) and, instead, begin to pay attention to the additives in our food and eliminate them from your diet. Consumer power is one way to fight back; you can hit the company's bottom line with your food choices and this will be a small but important step in signalling that change is needed in the way food is mass produced. The RYG programme is designed to include all-natural foods with no additives.

Pesticides

Pesticides (and fungicides) are the chemical compounds that farmers and food producers spray on crops to reduce the spread of bacteria or fungi, and to protect their produce from insects or rodents. You can be exposed to pesticides directly during their application, or indirectly through the water you drink, the dust in the air you breathe or as residues in the food you eat[17,18].

The World Health Organisation has collected data on over 100 pesticides and produced acceptable daily intake guidelines with the aim of ensuring the 'amount' of pesticides you are exposed to through eating food over your lifetime will not adversely affect your health. However, some of the chemical compounds found in these commonly used pesticides have been associated with short-term symptoms, such as headaches and nausea, as well as more severe conditions including certain kinds of cancer[18], hormone disruption[19], developmental delays in children[20] and neurological conditions like Parkinson's disease[21].

Effects of pesticide exposure may be more pronounced in children[20] as environmental toxins, including pesticide residues as mentioned previously, can be transferred to nursing children through breast milk[22] and crucially through the placenta to babies in the womb[23].

There seems to be an ongoing conflict between health authorities on the subject of pesticides. For example, in a review done by leading cancer researchers in 2015, scientists declared that glyphosate, a chemical found in many weedkillers, was genotoxic, meaning it causes DNA damage. It was also declared carcinogenic to animals and labelled a probable carcinogen to humans[24,25].

Glyphosate is best known as the main ingredient in Monsanto's Roundup brand along with many other products used by farmers and gardeners to kill weeds. The European Chemical Agency has dismissed the link between glyphosate and cancer but concedes that it can still cause serious eye damage after direct contact. But the plot thickens as the FDA in the USA has been forced to admit that their chemists found glyphosate levels at illegally high levels in honey products. A helpful analysis of the levels in your favourite food can be found in an article written by Carey Gillam "Not Just for Corn and Soy: A look at Glyphosate Use in Food Crops" [26].

At the time of writing, thousands of plaintiffs are suing Monsanto and have obtained millions of pages of internal Monsanto documents to support their claims, which they hope will show that glyphosate contributes to the development of non-Hodgkin's lymphoma and that Monsanto covered up the risks[27]. They will find it hard to show a direct link, but they are confident they have enough evidence.

Further research by independent scientists is required here. There is unnerving evidence from research that glyphosate residues in humans has dramatically increased, and the *Journal of the American Medical Association* published a study highlighting a dramatic increase in the amount of glyphosate found in human urine over the past 20 years[28]. A researcher in Dakota tested flour samples for glyphosate and found them all to have residues of the chemical[29]. In Europe glyphosate has been found widely in bread products[30]. Since glyphosate was introduced in 1974, 1.8 million tonnes has been used in US agriculture, 75% of this in the last 10 years.

Theoretically, organic foods should be free of residue, but a recent test of ten wines showed they all tested positive for glyphosate, even the organic ones[31]. Whilst the amount in the latter was lower, it clearly shows that spraying residue is contaminating organic vines nearby. Even German beer companies renowned for only using water, barley and hops to make their pure beer haven't escaped; a study by the Munich Environmental Institute found glyphosate in their 14 bestselling beers.

Glyphosate interestingly was patented by Monsanto as an antibiotic. Dr Stephanie Seneff at MIT has shown it disrupts the pathway in our gut bacteria that we rely on to produce amino acids that we are not able to make ourselves[32]. So most importantly glyphosate can disrupt our microbiome and we know how important that is for mental and physical health.

At the beginning of my journey, 18 years ago, which influenced me to write this book, I read the prescient book *Silent Spring* by Rachel Carson. In this book, she predicted the problems we are now facing, saying: "If we are going to live intimately with these chemicals, eating and drinking them, taking them into the marrow of our bones, we had better know something about their nature and power."

According to the Pesticide Action Network (PAN UK), about 60% of mass-produced fruit and vegetables contain pesticide residues in quantities that have been deemed 'safe' for human consumption (did you know bread, rice and flour can contain pesticide residue too?). However, PAN UK claims that nobody knows the long-term consequences of eating food that contains residues from various pesticides. So, what can you do?

The best way to reduce pesticides in your diet is to follow the Dirty Dozen, Clean Fifteen advice (see Chapter 2), and if possible grow your own fruit and vegetables. You could also consider buying organically grown foods, which have been found to contain around 30% of the pesticide residue of conventionally grown produce[33].

A family of five in Sweden participated in an experiment run by the Coop for the Swedish Environmental Research Institute. During the first week of the 21-day experiment, the family all ate a conventional diet and then each submitted a urine sample. Analysts found several insecticides, fungicides and plant growth regulators in these samples. Then, the family switched to an organic-only diet, including soaps and personal care items, for two weeks. During the organics phase, the researchers took daily urine samples. The results were dramatic: the pesticide loads in the family members' bodies dropped in ways that were observable after a single day, according to the report. And by the end of the two weeks, there was very little evidence of the pesticides and other compounds in their follow-up urine samples. Some may say this is only one family, and wasn't it great that the body did a good job at eliminating the chemicals, but wouldn't you want to reduce your chances of ingesting harmful chemicals in the first place?

Organisations like the Centre for Food Safety and True Food Network are working tirelessly to challenge potentially harmful problems in the food industry including "the spread of GMO foods, the profligate use of antibiotics in animal husbandry, the use of bee-killing pesticides and the production of engineered salmon". We can help this process by saying yes as much as possible to food that is organic and produced humanely[34].

Fish

We have seen that fish has been considered an integral part of a healthy diet. However, due to the rise in emissions from the combustion of fossil fuels, smelting and waste incineration, some seafood now contains dangerous levels of mercury. Around 95% of this is as methylmercury which cannot be removed by cleaning or cooking fish because it binds to proteins.

When I lived in the rainforests of Guyana, I saw the terrible effects of mercury poisoning. There were many small mining operations that used mercury to separate the gold from other residues. They would vaporise the mercury into the environment by heating the mixture. Once the mercury was in the environment it triggered Minimata disease, which can cause physical deformity.

While I was working in the Guyanese jungles I would meet children with no fingers on one hand, or with a club foot; they often lived near a mining site. One mother told me how she knew of parents "who would go as far as euthanasia when babies were born deformed"[35]. This is anecdotal, but the Amerindians told me that the rise in congenital deformities has coincided with the explosion in "bush mining".

Being exposed to mercury found in fish tissues has been found by some studies to increase your likelihood of developing cardiovascular diseases like atherosclerosis[36]. A good compromise, as suggested by the Food Standards Agency, is for you to eat species that are relatively low in mercury but high in omega-3. Omega-3 fish oil has been shown to reduce the risk of death from coronary heart disease or heart attack[37] and is associated with better cardiovascular health. Examples include Atlantic mackerel, salmon and cod. Bigger fish tend to contain higher levels of mercury so should not be consumed too often, eg swordfish, shark and fresh tuna[38].

Even this suggestion by the FDA is complicated by a study from the University of Albany which revealed that farmed salmon bought in Britain, Europe and North America contained significantly higher levels of organochlorine contaminants compared to wild salmon. These seem to be as a result of the feed given to farmed salmon[39].

However, we should remember that salmon has many positive effects: it is rich in omega-3 fatty acids and is a good source of protein and of vitamins and minerals (including potassium, selenium and vitamin B12). The NHS guidelines state that adults should be eating at least two portions of fish a week and one of these should be oily fish. Pregnant women, breastfeeding mothers and young children are advised to avoid fish high in mercury because they will be affected at lower concentrations, and mercury has been shown to have an adverse effect on a child's developing nervous system[40].

A great diagram from the BBC[41]:

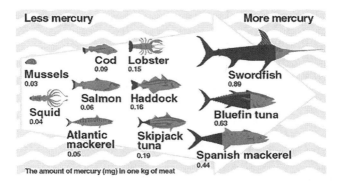

On top of the mercury issue, increasingly alarming ocean pollution means plastic wastes are now getting into fish and may end up on your plate. These microplastics are very dangerous as they accumulate in our bodies[42] and impose risks to our health. The incredible footage from the *Blue Planet* documentary series shows the alarming levels of plastic pollution in our oceans[43].

If this is incentive enough to cut all fish consumption, you can eat plant-based sources of omega-3 instead – such as flaxseed oil, chia seeds, walnuts and spinach. See www.ryghealth.com for veggie and vegan recipes.

We are what we drink

Water

Some water supplies contain fluoride added by local councils. It is a natural mineral that occurs in water and is known to protect our teeth, but there are concerns about its toxicity. *The Lancet* has recently classified it as a neurotoxin in the same category as arsenic and mercury[40]. Studies have revealed links between fluoride and ADHD[44] and there have been years of debate about the relationship between fluorinated water and cancer[45]. Recently, researchers at the University of Kent in an epidemiological study (this is a study of who, what and where) revealed that people living in areas of the UK with high fluoride levels were almost twice as likely to suffer from hypothyroidism (a condition that can cause weight gain and depression) than those who live in parts of the country with lower levels[46].

However, levels of fluoride in the UK for both ground water and that added by your water suppliers are below those quoted by The Fluoride Action Network (FAN) as being unsafe to drink. Some places in the world are not so lucky. In Arusha, Kenya, the local water has high levels of fluoride from the surrounding topography resulting in a high level of deformities in the local population. The Nasio Trust has raised funds to pipe in safe water. Apologies for the plug but they are always looking for volunteers to help with their projects, check out their website at: www.thenasiotrust.org.

If you're concerned about fluoride levels, it's a good idea for you to invest in a good filter, but be aware that not all filters remove fluoride, so choose carefully. Tap water in some countries is slightly chlorinated and the media has raised concerns about the chlorine levels in washed or ready to eat salads and that this may be a cancer risk[47]. The reference they used was sketchy and talks about chloroform, a good example of science being used to sensationalise!

Water bottles and plastic containers

It also makes sense to ditch your old water bottles and use a stainless steel or other BPA-free water bottle to reduce your exposure to BPA (bisphenol-a). This chemical, found in some polycarbonate plastic bottles, tableware, cutlery and food packaging (lining of food and drink cans), acts as an endocrine disruptor (a chemical that disrupts hormones[48]). A possible link between BPA exposure and certain kinds of cancers[49] (breast and prostate cancer) has been suggested, as well as increasing levels of infertility[50], early puberty[19] and the development of abnormal reproductive systems when tested on animals.

Presently the European Food Safety Authority (EFSA) regulates BPA and states that the current exposure for humans to BPA from food being in contact with plastic is considerably below the level required to cause an "appreciable risk to health". The level of BPA allowed in water bottles is now regulated.

So, have the authorities got the exposure covered? Even if not for the health concerns, it is worth cutting down on plastic use for environmental reasons. Plastic waste is right up there with climate change in important issues facing our planet.

Summing up

- Read labels on food, makeup and personal care products

- Avoid products that include trans fats in the ingredients

- Produce can have pesticide residue; organic produce tends to have less

- Choose fish low in mercury or get your beneficial omega-3 from plant sources like flaxseed

- Use a metal water bottle and filter your water when possible

Notes:

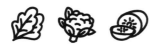

CHAPTER 9

External toxins

I n everyday life, considering and reducing your exposure to external toxins is a good idea. Here are a few examples and I am sure your gut bacteria will thank you for avoiding them.

Cookware

Earlier in this book, we looked at the merits of having a balanced diet for your microbiome, but it's not just what you eat that is important, it's how you cook your food too. You probably have a selection of non-stick pans in your kitchen cupboards, and while they might make washing-up easier, some people are concerned that the substance might be carcinogenic. Is this true?

The simple answer is not necessarily. Non-stick pans in the past used to use the substance perfluorooctanoic acid (PFOA), which has since been deemed by the International Agency for Research on Cancer

(IARC) (part of the World Health Organisation) to be 'possibly carcinogenic to humans'. The primary route for human exposure was through drinking water[1,2], but since 2016 the use of PFOA has been phased out and most non-stick pans are now coated with the substance polytetrafluoroethylene (PTFE, also known as Teflon). PTFE is not suspected of causing cancer as long as it isn't heated to ridiculously high temperatures (ie heating the pan to high temperatures with nothing in it) as possibly carcinogenic fumes may then be released[3]. If you're still worried, get rid of your old non-stick pans and switch to stainless steel or cast iron pans, which do not contain PTFE.

Radiation

Since mobile phones were introduced, there has been uncertainty around possible health risks. In today's technical, ever connected world, what does the current evidence say?

Mobile phones: do they cause cancer?

Mobiles and other devices emit radio-frequency radiation, a type of electromagnetic field radiation. Numerous studies have been conducted to assess the possible risk that this type of radiation could have on health, and so far there are no indications of a link with cancer [4-6]. Unlike high-energy (ionising) radiation, there is no proof that radio frequency radiation damages DNA or cells directly.

However, in 2011 the IARC classified electrical devices as 'possibly' carcinogenic[4,5] to humans and research continues to fully assess the potential effects of mobile phone use. Studies in the past on animals have shown no increased cancer risk for long-term exposure to radio-frequency fields. But the IARC states we can only say that regularly using devices for up to ten years does not seem to cause cancer as mobile devices have only been widely available since the 1990s, and there are no comprehensive studies to investigate the long-term effects of mobile phones.

Some studies (not accepted by the mobile industry) are beginning to emerge that are asserting that the warning from the WHO that EMF radiation is a possible human carcinogen is well founded. Dr Thomas Rau, medical director of the renowned Paracelsus Clinic in Switzerland, states that EMFs from wireless networks and mobile phones can cause cancer, ADD (Attention Deficit Disorder), heart arrhythmias, insomnia and Parkinson's disease. The European Academy for Environmental Medicine agrees, reporting that EMF radiation is linked to cancer, insomnia and mental health disorders. Ulrich Warnke, an internationally esteemed professor from the University of Saarland, asserts that EMF radiation from light transmitters can cause disruption of the body's nitrogen monoxide system, which keeps cells healthy and regulates gene expression.

A study conducted by the National Institute of Health's National Toxicology Programme provided a definitive link between 2G/3G mobile phone radiation and heart and brain cancer in rats. Researchers cited "clear evidence of carcinogenicity" [7]. An additional study conducted at the Rammazzini Institute for Environmental Policy reinforced the results of the NTP study. Both showed a statistically significant increase in rare malignancies – the very same malignancies found in population studies of human mobile phone users. Finally, recent research shows that pregnant women exposed to the highest levels of EMF radiation are 48% more likely to lose their babies than women exposed to the lowest amount [8].

EMF Scientists – an alliance of 220 researchers and doctors from 42 different countries – is currently appealing to the UN to ask the WHO to develop stricter EMF guidelines, and to better educate the public as to the risks. All of these studies need more investigation as to the impact on human health.

What can you do?

You can minimise EMF radiation exposure with some common sense precautions, such as: keeping mobile phones away from the body, turning wifi off when not in use, and keeping devices in airplane mode when you are not using them. Whenever possible, use speakerphones or a hands-free headset, and keep conversations brief, or text or even use a landline.

So, despite our overwhelming reliance on these devices, while research continues on the link between the radiation emitted and cancer, it might be a good idea to limit mobile phone use, especially in your children. Even if researchers do provide definitive evidence of no cancer risk, I'm still a huge advocate for reducing screen time on devices just in case they do have long-term consequences for our mental health. Too often, we find ourselves forgetting the present moment because we are staring down at screens. Putting phones away is important for spending quality time with family, and, as discussed later, reducing screen time before bed can improve sleep, which reduces inflammation and nurtures the health of your microbiome.

If you want to limit your exposure to mobile phone radiation, the UK charity Mobilewise makes the following recommendations:

- Text instead of calling

- Don't sleep next to a mobile phone

- Use a headset and carry your phone in a bag rather than a pocket

- Ration children's use of mobiles (so they don't get the habit – my advice)

Blue light

'Blue light' emitted from the screens of your hand-held devices can interfere with your sleep hormones and alertness[9] by inhibiting the production of the sleep hormone melatonin[10]. Blue light regulates the body's circadian rhythm, so by exposing yourself to blue light at times when you naturally wouldn't (ie the evenings and at night) you fool your body into thinking it is really still day when it is night[11]. This makes it harder for you to nod off and affects the quality of your sleep.

According to the Harvard Medical School's advice, you can reduce the impact blue light has on your sleep patterns, and ultimately your health, by:

- Getting as much natural light as you can during the day[12]

- Try to avoid looking at screens from two to three hours before bed

- Using dim red lights for night lights as they have the least power to shift your circadian rhythm

A time bomb?

I mention the following research hesitantly because further studies are needed.

Laptops and tablets

One study has shown that radiation produced by wifi enabled laptops has been shown to have negative effects on human sperm quality in the lab[13]. More work is needed to see if this decline in quality occurs in sperm still within the testes. The process of producing sperm – spermatogenesis – occurs optimally at temperatures just below human body temperature[14]. So, given that laptops can emit heat, and that radiation produced by these devices may lower sperm quality, you could avoid the potential risk by simply not putting it on your lap and using a desk.

Some people suffer from EMF hypersensitivity where symptoms such as nausea, fainting, dizziness, headaches, heart palpitations, tinnitus and sleep disorders can occur. Reduction in the use of electronic devices can go some way towards alleviating a person's exposure to EMFs. Equally, removing devices from the bedroom has been shown to be beneficial too. To determine levels of EMFs you can use a radio frequency meter which will analyse the possible radiation exposure from wifi, mobile phones etc in your home. For more information, visit http://www.es-uk.info/.

Home hazards

Cleaning products: how clean do you need to be?

Most of us have cupboards crammed full of polish and disinfectants, and whilst cleanliness is important, the ingredients in many of these products are in fact highly toxic. Some of the chemicals they contain can cause breathing problems, burns and eye irritation.

We are being told repeatedly (and often to our relief!) that too much household cleaning is bad for us, but is there any truth to these stories? The answer is yes: some cleaning products are literally bursting with toxins.

Bleach is probably the worst culprit, and whilst it might leave the toilet fresh and your surfaces sparkling, it is something that should be used sparingly and in well-ventilated areas. New research from the French National Institute of Medical Research revealed that people who inhaled fumes from bleach and other powerful cleaning products had up to a 32% increased risk of developing chronic obstructive pulmonary disease (COPD)[15], a debilitating lung condition. A separate study also suggests that bleach used for domestic cleaning could be linked with non-allergic asthma[16].

Another study, this time by the Centre for Environment and Health in Belgium, claimed that schoolchildren living in homes where bleach was used on a regular basis had a significantly increased risk of coming down with flu, pneumonia and tonsillitis[17]. There was also a study done on children with leukaemia that showed they had higher concentrations of two common pesticides found in household cleaners (DETP and DEDTP) in their urine compared to healthy children. Researchers stated this does not show the cleaners caused the cancer, but it signifies a health hazard that needs to be investigated[18].

Phthalates are a group of chemicals that have been linked to asthma, ADHD, breast cancer, male infertility issues and type 2 diabetes. They are frequently found in air fresheners, washing-up liquid and wipes. Researchers from the University of Adelaide revealed a potential association between phthalate exposure and chronic disease prevalence, including cardiovascular disease[19]. Phthalates are also found in household plastics, tin foil and cling film. A recent study of 3,000 American children aged between 6 and 19 showed that those who had been exposed to phthalates had higher blood pressure than those who had not[20].

However, the last two are both epidemiological studies and so do not support the causation argument. In other words, we cannot say irrefutably that phthalates cause these health problems, and several government scientific agencies and the Centre for Disease Control and Prevention have concluded that the exposure for humans was "significantly lower than any level of concern set by regulatory agencies".

So again, a conflicting set of information. I would suggest if a product says it contains 'parfum' or 'fragrance', there is a good chance it contains phthalates. So, instead opt for labels with the descriptions 'phthalate-free', 'no synthetic fragrance' or those scented with only essential oils.

Triclosan is found in most washing-up liquids and antibacterial hand soaps. This chemical can cause skin irritation, and animal studies have shown it to be an endocrine (hormone) disrupter[21,22] although further research is needed to see if these findings are transferrable to humans. The use of this broad-spectrum antimicrobial agent is also creating triclosan-resistant bacteria[23]. The European Commission restricts the use of triclosan, but you will still find it in many household products.

While research continues on rats to try to determine the effects of triclosan on humans, if you are concerned it may be worth avoiding products containing it, especially if you are breastfeeding or pregnant[24]. Look out for triclosan (TSC) and triclocarban (TCC) on the labels, and instead of using antibacterial soaps use plain soap, warm water and thorough washing.

Note: Other chemicals that should be used with caution because they can cause skin or eye irritation, include:

- Quarternary ammonium compounds or 'Quats'

- 2-Butoxyethanol

- Chlorine

- Sodium hydroxide

Chemical-free cleaning

If you are a born 'neat freak', don't despair – you can still have a clean home if you don't use the products mentioned above to excess. And if you decide you want to eliminate these possible chemicals further, why not opt for some of the cleaning materials used by previous generations? Try these for a start:

- **Vinegar** is free from toxins and because it has such a high acid content it can combat even the toughest bacteria. Fill the bath with warm water and add four cups of vinegar, and then drain after three hours for a sparkling tub. Or add a cup to your toilet and leave it overnight before flushing for a germ-free loo.

- **Bicarbonate of soda** is another natural cleaning agent – its alkalinity means it can dissolve grime and add sparkle to stained cups and cloths. You could make your own in a spray bottle and add essential oils for an aromatherapy hit. It is also great for cleaning carpets. Just sprinkle it on and leave overnight before vacuuming up.

Personal care products: how beautiful?

Cosmetics and skincare

A recent survey by the non-profit Environmental Working Group (EWG) in the USA revealed that the average woman applies 126 chemicals to her skin every day, and that's usually before breakfast! While our cherished beauty products might make us look good and smell fantastic, the long-term effects on our bodies aren't nearly so brilliant.

It is important to be aware of exactly what you are putting on to your body. Two of the major chemicals to try and avoid are parabens – antimicrobial additives which can be found in up to 85% of beauty and personal care products – and again, phthalates. Like BPA and certain pesticides, parabens and phthalates can act as endocrine disruptors when present in high quantities[25]. They are also found in shampoos, shower gels, and makeup.

You may be thinking that the small doses found in skincare and makeup products are not high enough to be damaging to our health, but given that these chemicals appear to be so ubiquitous, is it even impossible to avoid them altogether? You can always check the label for phthalate- and paraben-free alternatives and steer clear of anything containing DBP, DEP, DEHP, BzBP, 'fragrance' or 'parfum'.

Makeup

It is important to be aware of what you are putting on to your skin. Our skin is our largest organ and anything we put on it could potentially be absorbed directly into our bloodstream.

Mascara

You might crave long lashes, but did you know that most mascara has a shelf life of just four months? Yet a recent report commissioned by an eye hospital group revealed that some British women are using the same eye wand for up to ten years. Now if that's not a breeding ground for bacteria, what is? Using out of date products and keeping eye makeup on for too long can cause serious eye infections, as can sharing pencils and not keeping brushes and curlers clean.

Nail varnish

For most of us, getting our nails done is a real treat. Recently, however, there has been a lot of concern in the media fuelled by Dr Thu Quach at Stanford University[26] who looked at the so-called toxic trio that can be found in some nail polishes. These are toluene, which creates a smooth finish – this chemical, when inhaled, has been found in some studies to affect the nervous system; formaldehyde, which is a nail-hardening agent and has been classified by the International Agency for Research on Cancer as a known carcinogen[27]; and dibutyl phthalate, which has been linked to reproductive problems in some animal studies[28].

However, before you panic, acceptable amounts of these chemicals is being debated. It seems unlikely that the amounts present in these products are high enough to cause these effects[29]. Even so, it is best to put your varnish on outside and, if you're visiting a salon, make sure it is well ventilated. If you're still concerned, why not use a nail varnish brand which doesn't use these chemicals, like Ondine, a company that makes varnishes from natural pigments such as resin and water?

Lipstick

Many lipsticks contain synthetic colours, which are made from coal tar. These can cause skin sensitivity, or as one study terms it 'cosmetic dermatitis'[30] and have been linked to some cancers[31]. Lipstick, foundation and eye makeup can also contain elements such as arsenic, mercury and lead which can interfere with the immune, reproductive and nervous systems. They are banned in cosmetics in the EU but may be present at very small levels as contaminants[32] and apparently some women may accidentally consume up to 5kg of lipstick in their lifetime!

It is certainly possible to avoid coal tar derivatives if you wish: just check the label and opt for brands that don't use synthetic colours.

Deodorants

It is well known that spray-on deodorants can cause health problems; Allergy UK makes a point of warning people that the aerosols can exacerbate asthma, eczema and rhinitis.

There is also some speculation amongst the medical community that the aluminium found in antiperspirants might be able to enter your cells and disrupt them, causing cancer[33]. However, for the moment, researchers say there is no proven link between deodorants and breast cancer[34].

The pores under our arms are specifically designed to expel sweat and toxins, but as there's no conclusive evidence to suggest that you need to ditch the deodorant, to put any concerns you may have at bay you could try:

- Putting on sprays with the windows open

- Opt for aluminium-free deodorant

- Buying salt crystal block deodorants

Synthetic scents

These scents might make our bodies and homes smell sweet, but they can contain allergens and irritants which cause unhealthy effects such as respiratory difficulties, migraine headaches, skin, neurological, cognitive, immune, cardiovascular and musculoskeletal issues, and most relevantly for this book, gastrointestinal problems[35]. As mentioned above under phthalates, opt for 'phthalate-free', 'no synthetic fragrance' or even try essential oils to make your home smell fresh. For more information on these chemicals and where you might find them, visit www.safecosmetics.org.uk.

Personal care products: sun cream

We all need some exposure to the sun for vitamin D production. Indeed, in the UK lack of sunlight exposure is a major cause of vitamin D deficiency (discussed further in Chapter 10). Cancer Research UK recommends exposure to the sun before 11am and after 3pm for at least 20 to 30 minutes whenever you can, to benefit from the sun's influence on vitamin D production, while avoiding the most damaging rays at midday.

That said, it's worth bearing in mind that not all sun lotions are as effective as you might think. Research has revealed that some high street brands might prevent you from getting burnt, but they don't protect you from the UV damage that can cause skin cancer. Check the details before you buy, and that they are free from skincare nasties like oxybenzone and homosalate that are known hormone disruptors. Look for zinc or titanium dioxide-based creams without parabens, phthalates or artificial fragrances. Cancer Research UK is now advising people that the best way to protect themselves from the sun's more damaging rays is by wearing hats and covering up.

Summing up

- Switch off your laptop and mobile as often as you can or turn off wifi when not in use

- Look at natural alternatives when it comes to cleaning and cosmetics

- Avoid synthetic sprays and fragrances; opt for essential oils instead, for the sake of your guts!

Notes:

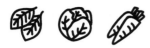

CHAPTER 10

It is your choice

So far we've explored the importance of the gut bacteria, eating well, regular exercise, good mental health, reducing inflammation, and the influence of toxins and drugs on mental and physical wellbeing. If it isn't already clear, the overall message is simple: you can look after your health by making a few basic lifestyle choices and our bodies are amazing at detoxifying if given the chance.

Unfortunately, with the mind-blowing number of health myths out there nowadays (not to mention the ever changing government guidelines), it's often hard to work out precisely what those lifestyle choices are. Who knows how many people have subjected themselves to near starvation trying to emulate the latest celebrity diet?

With so much misinformation and conflicting research, you might be unsure what to believe. As ever, my recommendation is to consider the evidence carefully and trust your gut reaction (no pun intended). You really do have the power to make the right decisions for your health, the trick is to listen to your body's needs and adjust your habits accordingly. This chapter is intended to give you the confidence to make sensible, informed choices that will help you achieve a healthier body and a happier mind.

The conventional vs the functional approach

Currently, diagnoses made by doctors, especially in mental health, are based on studies and criteria that academics work hard to provide. Drugs are tested against placebos, an existing treatment, and use double blind trials (neither the patients nor the researchers know who is getting a placebo and who is getting the treatment) to add to the rigour of the process.

However, in my eyes (and in the eyes of the rapidly growing community of functional medical practitioners encouraged and educated by the Institute of Functional Medicine) this is not the whole story and not the best way of approaching the problem at hand.

If health were like a rainforest, handing people a specific diagnosis and a treatment targeted at that specific problem (but nothing else) is like cutting down one diseased tree while ignoring that the rest of the jungle is sick too. Often, we are prescribed one drug for depression, another for indigestion and yet another for constipation, when these are all symptoms of a body in disarray. Your body is like the rainforest and needs to be treated as a whole and nurtured to bring it back to full health with optimum diversity.

While you may feel better when taking drugs, the reality is that this may be masking the fact that your body is not in a healthy state. A functional medicine approach would look at the underlying cause to treat the physiological damage and then work with your body systems (as a whole) to help them heal. All this is done while focusing on your symptoms to see what helps them to improve[1].

To make this clearer, here is a practical example of the current approach. If you are suffering from acid reflux you may be prescribed acid-blocking drugs. While this will give temporary relief in the short term, in the long term these drugs may disrupt your gut microbiome and allow pathogenic bacteria to flourish. Conventional medicine will then try to clear up these pathogenic bacteria with antibiotics, restarting the vicious cycle of disease-drug-disease all over again.

Functional medicine, on the other hand, takes a more considered and often more effective approach. For instance, conventional medical practitioners are likely to tackle a *C. difficile* infection (a pathogenic bacterium that infects the bowels and causes diarrhoea) by prescribing antibiotics – an intervention only thought to be effective in 26% of cases. Functional medicine practitioners have tackled this problem directly and opted for a faecal transplant (in simplistic terms giving a sick patient faecal matter from a healthy person), a treatment shown to be effective in 96% of cases[2]. This is functional medicine at its best – not using drugs to mask symptoms in the short term but instead rebalancing gut bacteria and avoiding long-term damage.

Success with faecal transplants has been seen in other areas as well. Doctors did a faecal microbial transplant in an attempt to alleviate the symptoms and hopefully cure type 2 diabetes[3] and autism[4]. In both these conditions the patients showed abnormal organisms in their gut and the faecal transplant restored the balance of their gut bacteria, and patients experienced a dramatic improvement in their condition. Sadly, at the moment, faecal transplants are not cheap, but I am hopeful that with the long-term cost benefits to our health and health services, and more research, they will become the norm to rebalance our bodies.

I hope it is becoming clear that[5] a wide array of mental and physical problems – from mental health conditions and hormonal imbalances to immune conditions and poor sleep – may, in fact, arise due to a dysfunction of the gut and its microbiome. Conventional doctors are likely to give patients suffering from such ailments a diagnosis and attempt to treat with drugs and/or therapy. Functional medicine practitioners, in contrast, do not believe formal diagnosis is the priority. Instead, they would recommend assessing the state of the body (eg through functional tests) and attempting to fix any obvious imbalances, such as microbial imbalance, before turning to medication.

Functional medicine boils down to a very simple idea: look at your body as a whole, make changes to promote balance across all body systems, and then, if needed, combine with formal treatments such as therapy or appropriate medication. It is common sense, really.

Information is power

When it comes to making positive choices, in any walk of life, it pays to be informed. With that in mind, let's have a look at some key areas of debate in the field of physical and mental health. Hopefully, this will arm you with the information you need to exercise your power to choose effectively and, ultimately, achieve your health goals.

The True Health Initiative, a group of 400 nutrition experts I mentioned earlier in the book, recommend that people wanting to look after their health follow a basic set of nutritional guidelines: eat local, mostly plant-based non-refined foods, drink mostly water, and some tea and coffee. These guys are not trying to sell a specific way of eating (eg veganism, ketogenic diets, paleo etc) and promising miraculous results, they're just trying to simplify what it means to eat well. This is the same approach as the *Reset Your Gut* programme.

Will eating healthily lead to an eating disorder?

We are often told we shouldn't focus too much on our diet and weight, and with the rates of eating disorders at an all-time high, the fear that obsessing too much over our waistlines will have awful consequences for our mental health is entirely understandable. But does that mean we should stop making an effort to stay healthy altogether?

There have been various articles in the popular press over the last few years about the dangers of 'orthorexia' – an eating disorder characterised by an obsessive desire to 'live cleanly'. People with this condition can become so fixated on clean living (eating healthily, exercising regularly etc) that they begin to avoid social situations for fear of it stopping them achieving their health goals and, paradoxically, to deprive their bodies of certain nutrients by avoiding 'bad' foods[6].

While I understand the concern over lifestyle habits becoming overly restrictive, I believe it is important to stress that eating well does *not* make you orthorexic. What's more, the existence of the term orthorexia – and the associated stigma – is making it increasingly difficult for people to make positive changes to their lifestyles. I have witnessed patients' attempts to follow a Mediterranean diet to reduce inflammation and improve their mental health, only to have 'helpful' friends destabilise their efforts by accusing them of being on the verge of developing orthorexia. Simple lifestyle changes within an unsupportive environment can be very tough and totally unfair on people trying to look after themselves better by improving their daily habits.

Do we need to count calories to lose weight?

Obesity is a very serious health issue. New research from The Organisation for Economic Cooperation and Development (OECD) has revealed that the UK is now the most obese nation in Western Europe, as almost 30% of British adults now have a BMI of 30 (the official definition of obesity) or above. By 2030, the OECD predicts that 35% of the country's adults will be obese[7].

Obesity is a major risk factor for many non-communicable diseases and it's essential that you make an effort to maintain a healthy weight. Sadly, the messages on how best to lose weight can be exceptionally confusing. One question in particular keeps popping up: do you need to count calories to shed those extra kilos/pounds?

You'll be happy to hear, the answer in this case is a definite **no**.

The idea that dieting and weight loss is wholly dependent on 'calories in vs calories out' was first promoted in the 1950s by a sugar industry hell bent on turning high-fat foods into the diet demon and replacing them with low-fat, sugar-filled alternatives (see below). Indeed, this was, and sadly is, the central premise for many weight-loss programmes.

However, it is now widely accepted that calorie counting is outdated, misleading and an exceptionally poor guide to nutrition. Nutritional therapist Amelia Freer stresses that peoples' calorie needs can vary according to their age, sleep quality, gut health, and levels of activity, so counting them will never be very accurate[8]. Your priority should be listening to your body and eating primarily wholefoods that leave you feeling satisfied and energised.

Not only that, but there is increasing evidence that all calories were *not,* in fact, created equal. For instance, there is an enormous difference between the calories in a sugar-sweetened drink and those in wholefoods such as fruits and starchy vegetables. In the US, one court is considering introducing a warning label on sugar-sweetened drinks following an investigation in which researchers agreed that they "were uniquely harmful to human health"[9]. A healthy diet consisting of minimally processed wholegrains, fruit, vegetables and healthy fats – regardless of their calorific score – is definitely better for you than one of processed foods, sugar and junk, regardless of their caloric value.

Does healthy eating mean avoiding all sugars?

In recent years, sugar has been blamed for just about everything. From tooth decay and hyperactivity, to weight gain and type 2 diabetes – sugar really is the nutritional pitfall of this generation. The evidence against the sweet stuff has been building for quite some time. It emerged recently that in 1967 the sugar industry sat on a report linking sucrose to heart disease and some cancers, and the results were never published[10].

When the truth began to emerge about sugar effects on our health, Coca-Cola created the Global Energy Balance Network and recruited Sense about Science and the University of Colorado Medical School to promote the idea that sugar was not the problem; it was a misbalance in energy and people just needed to exercise. This notion has been debunked, and to their credit the Colorado Med School handed back the funding they were given by Coca-Cola.

But do you have to stop eating sugar completely? Of course not! While it's probably best to avoid the sweet stuff when it's found in packaged biscuits, cakes and other processed food, you can still indulge your sweet tooth without feeling guilty. Why not grab a piece of fruit, a few dates or a couple of pieces of dark chocolate? These are all great ways of getting that sweet taste without worrying about the long-term consequences to your health!

Dark chocolate may not be labelled as a 'super food' but it does have some health benefits due its high cacao profile. The flavonoids and polyphenols found in cacao are antioxidants that can reduce oxidative stress in the body, which can ultimately contribute to cancer prevention[11]. Regular chocolate consumption has also been shown to reduce blood pressure and prevent cardiovascular diseases[12] although the protective effects of chocolate were not observed with more than one serving, so eating more chocolate sadly won't help more. A trial in 2018 at Loma Linda University showed that "consumption of dark chocolate (70% cacao) reduced stress and inflammation". Sounds like a fun study to do, sign me up!

Flavonoids really are a wonder chemical. Not only are they thought to contribute to improving your cognitive processes by aiding memory and learning[13] but also to reducing insulin resistance and hypertension[14]. Finally, dark chocolate is also packed with beneficial minerals and vitamins such as potassium, iron, zinc and calcium.

That being said, before you rush out and bulk buy your favourite chocolate, check the label. Dark chocolate, preferably 70% or above, is the most likely to give you the above health benefits, while the average bar of milk chocolate (containing around 110g of sugar) has almost no nutritional value[15].

Should we avoid fizzy drinks? Are diet drinks a better option?

It is, of course, your choice, but the evidence against sugary drinks is pretty conclusive due to their high sugar content and vastly documented links to obesity[16-18], heart disease[19,20] and type 2 diabetes[21]. A study by the American Heart Association revealed that regular consumption of these drinks has been linked to 130,000 new cases of diabetes in the USA over a ten-year period[22]. On top of that, researchers at the University of Minnesota claim that drinking just two of these beverages a week could double your risk of pancreatic cancer[23], while another study revealed that consuming 25% or more of your daily calories from added sugar can triple your risk of heart disease[24].

Diet fizzy drinks, in contrast, are drinks that contain artificial sweeteners instead of sugar to help you reduce your intake while still satisfying your sweet tooth. But are they any better for your health? Unfortunately, this is a very controversial area of research and a clear answer to this question is yet to emerge.

Researchers at the University of Texas's Health Science Centre found that people who drank a diet fizzy drink every day saw their waistlines expand by an average of three inches over a 10-year period. The researchers weren't entirely sure why this happened, but they suggested it might be due to artificial sweeteners making people hungrier and therefore eating more. A study by researchers at the Weizmann Institute of Science in Rehovot, Israel, suggested that there is a link between the consumption of artificial sweeteners and glucose intolerance, and that the link may be to do with alterations to our friends in the gut microbiome[25].

The study was predominantly carried out on mice, with only a small study on healthy humans showing an association between artificial sweetener intake and glucose intolerance, so further investigation is definitely required. There is evidence that common sweeteners such as sucralose, acesulfame-K and aspartame[26] have a complex impact on our microbiome and, as such, it may be to best to avoid foods sweetened with these if possible.

Another study goes further and says artificial sweeteners "are far from helping to solve the global obesity crisis". It stated that due to "the composition of low nutrient density and food additives and consumption patterns (ie potential promotion of sweet taste preference), and environmental impact (misuse of natural resources, pollution, or ecotoxicity) it makes sweeteners a potential risk factor for highly prevalent chronic diseases"[27]. You see how complicated academic research can appear!

Gluten

If sugar is now considered to be the source of all dietary evil, gluten would probably win second place. Indeed, so great is the stigma surrounding it that the American chat show host Jimmy Kimmel jokingly said it had become comparable to satanism in Los Angeles. For Hollywood A-Listers, following a gluten-free diet is probably as standard as employing a personal trainer and doing yoga. Even in the UK, many people are jumping on the bandwagon with 8% of people now identifying as avoiding gluten as part of a healthy lifestyle. The demand for gluten-free products is growing exponentially, with the 'free-from' market (responsible for the sale of a wide array of gluten-free and dairy-free products) at a net worth of £531m at last estimates.

What is gluten?

Gluten is made up of two different proteins: giadin and glutenin. It helps foods maintain their shape and can be found not just in wheat, barley and rye but in many processed foods and ingredients, including soy, gravy granules and packet soups too.

Why is it bad?

Critics of gluten – and there are many – claim that humans simply don't have the right enzymes needed to break down gluten properly, causing the immune system to attack it as an invader. This is certainly true for the 1% of the population who have coeliac disease, an autoimmune illness caused by a reaction to gluten, resulting in inflammation and symptoms such as bloating, diarrhoea, nausea, fatigue, anaemia and weight loss[28].

Interestingly, an increasing number of people are now being diagnosed with gluten intolerance or non-coeliac gluten sensitivity. This means they don't experience inflammation per se but nonetheless experience a negative reaction when they consume gluten[29]. There is no mainstream diagnostic test available for this condition, but sufferers find that cutting out gluten greatly improves their symptoms (see below).

Are you gluten intolerant?

If you're not sure whether gluten is causing your uncomfortable digestive issues, why not ask yourself if you are suffering from any of the lesser known side effects of a gluten intolerance[28]. These are:

- Diarrhoea

- Weight loss

- Depression and fatigue

- Iron deficiency

- Anaemia

- Neurological conditions, brain fog and headaches

- Vitamin D deficiency

- Sleepiness/tired after eating gluten

If you regularly experience any of these symptoms after eating gluten, it might be worth temporarily eliminating it from your diet (ie for a month or so like the RYG programme) and seeing if it helps. Then, when you later reintroduce it back into your diet, see whether the problems persist. Some people will only have a slight sensitivity and you may not need to cut it out entirely, although it might be worth going easy on the pizza and cake! It is also worth bearing in mind that new research from the University of Oslo has revealed that intolerance to fructans (the sugar chains found in wheat, barley and rye) can present with similar symptoms to gluten sensitivity[30].

Just a fad?

The fact that fashion retailer Zara produced a t-shirt emblazoned with the slogan *'Are you gluten free?'* is perhaps a sign of just how trendy avoiding gluten has become. These controversial tops were quickly discontinued after a deluge of customer complaints, many claiming that it trivialised an important health problem.

And I believe they had a point.

Both my daughter and I find gluten hard to stomach, even just indulging in pizza can result in immediate diarrhoea, headache and a rash. A friend, on returning from a week in an expensive medical clinic and knowing of our challenge, relayed the following advice from the expert there: "Most people are only intolerant and can eat gluten from time to time. And, let's face it, it's bad form and boorish to avoid it when being fed at other people's houses!"

This advice is acceptable as you may be able to tolerate a small amount from time to time, but the clinic also told a lady who said that gluten made her feel unwell that: "People who don't eat what is put in front of them on social occasions and fussed about food in general often developed neurosis in other areas that in turn affects self-confidence, happiness, self-worth and the ability to get on with peers." This is extraordinary advice and a good example of conventional medicine getting it seriously wrong, a clear case of someone trying to eat healthily but being told they had orthorexia.

I do object to the idea that those who choose not to eat gluten because it makes them feel rubbish are being told it is 'quite unnecessary' and 'was likely to lead to mental instability'. As my 16-year-old daughter said when she read what the clinic doctor had said: "Does that mean if I refuse pudding I will lose confidence? BS! It means I am choosing to not feel unwell. What happened to free choice?"

One study in America claimed that adopting a gluten-free diet could potentially do more damage to your heart as it generally equates to eating less wholegrains which are good for cardiac health[31]. There is also anecdotal evidence to suggest that eating gluten-free foods can have a negative effect on your waistline as they tend to contain more fat to give them more texture; however, if you eat non-gluten wholegrains and fresh produce both these objections are irrelevant.

I have no doubt the effects of gluten will continue to be contested but, as always, my advice is simply to follow your gut. If it makes you feel rubbish, cut it out.

Vaccines

Vaccines are, of course, an exceptionally controversial topic and it was for that reason that I seriously considered skipping this section entirely. However, to ignore the confusion that surrounds vaccines (partly due to inaccurate media coverage) is to ignore one of the biggest public health issues of this generation.

All vaccines come with their own health risks, as listed in the side effect documents provided when you have the vaccine. Personally, I think you must balance up the risk of complications from the vaccine against the risk of the thing you are being vaccinated against. Without vaccines, there is no doubt that people would still be dying from dangerous infections like polio, diphtheria and whooping cough. Interestingly, it has been shown that the efficacy of vaccines is influenced by the gut microbiome, so a healthy composition of intestinal microbiome contributes to strong immunity. This again emphasises the importance of a healthy diet[32].

I would say I am sceptical of the pharmaceutical industry's motives for introducing so many new vaccines, especially for children, but in some countries including Canada and the US, vaccines are made mandatory for children to attend school[33]. Sweden has banned mandatory vaccinations citing "serious health concerns" and the fact that it "violates a citizen's right to choose their own health care". Yet, although Sweden's programme is voluntary, the vast majority of children are still vaccinated.

To vaccinate or not to vaccinate? That is the question

Ultimately, in the UK it is still your choice. An important consideration is the concept of herd immunity, a form of indirect protection from infectious disease that occurs when a large percentage of a population has become immune to an infection, thereby providing a measure of protection for individuals who are not.

I wish I had a more clear-cut answer – hopefully further research will reveal one in time. I think it is important to recognise the controversy and also recognise that there is a place for evidence-based medicine guidelines, as any doctor will tell you when they have witnessed children die from a disease that a vaccine might have prevented.

Are your genes your destiny?

Conventional medicine has previously taken the view that your genetic makeup dictates who you are and what diseases you will end up developing, and that there's very little you can do (except medicate if it turns up.). However, in this book I have shown again and again how lifestyle choice can affect your health outcomes, but where there is a definite genetic condition it is best that functional medicine works in conjunction with the options drugs have given us to reduce symptoms.

A cardiologist who is very keen to implement lifestyle solutions gave me a great example. Her patient had a genetic condition that is characterised by high cholesterol levels and had suffered two strokes and needed a quadruple bypass. Even after seriously changing his lifestyle and losing a significant amount of weight, his cholesterol was high. In this case she felt there was a place for prescribing statins and to work hand in hand with the lifestyle changes in the hope that fewer drugs would be required.

So, ultimately, your health outcome is about your choices. While there are too many health debates to cover them all, I hope this chapter has given you at least some confidence to think beyond the hearsay and to start making your own informed decisions. If in doubt, just remember:

Summing up

- It's your body, and your call

- Always investigate further if you're unsure

- You are in charge! Listen to your body

- You do not necessarily need to count calories to lose weight

- Use scientific evidence to make informed choices suitable for your body's needs

- Vaccine efficacy is influenced by the balance of your gut bacteria

Notes:

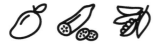

CHAPTER 11

Testing...testing... testing

If you're reading this book, you're already committing to making your health a priority. Hopefully, after the past few chapters, you're now starting to realise the importance of eating well, exercising regularly, limiting your stress levels and exposure to environmental toxins – all good aims if you want to maximise your mental and physical wellbeing.

But what after doing all this you still feel rubbish?

If you have *Reset Your Gut*, got more sleep and started exercising regularly, what next? I would encourage you to get functional health tests to work out the state of your body: to identify your nutritional deficiencies and what specifically you need to pay attention to in your busy life. Some doctors will be reluctant to order these tests and may say they are not necessary, but if this is the case, you can always reach out to a functional medicine practitioner and get help elsewhere.

I suggest these tests after having done the RYG programme for purely economic reasons, as you may find you don't need them at all. Whilst there is an argument that testing before the course would enable you to target specific minerals or vitamins, the tests are not cheap, and paying attention to rebalancing your microbiome may be all you need to have a healthier body and a happier mind.

We know from Chapter 1 there is a growing body of evidence about the connection between mental health and physical health and the state of your gut. Below are a few of the physical tests I would encourage you to consider if you are diagnosed with a mental or physical illness and prescribed talking therapies and/or drugs. Lifelong medication is not a given if you can find the root cause (eg nutrient deficiencies, physiological imbalances etc) and fix them yourself.

Some of the following tests may cost you money as they are not freely available from the NHS. However, I am hopeful that the ever increasing number of functional medicine practitioners means these tests will eventually become readily available. It's definitely something worth campaigning for.

Your gut

Here are tests related to your gut health that you might want to consider.

Gut bacteria profiling

Doctors Data, Functional DX, Genova Diagnostics[1] and others offer profiling of the bacteria in your gut. If you suffer from indigestion, gastritis, heartburn, bloating, reflux, nausea or decreased appetite, it could be worth considering these tests, which can be performed by testing your stools.

Your individual results, which show the diversity of your gut microbiome, are compared to the patterns seen in patients with clinical conditions such as IBS. They can also tell you whether you are carrying parasites or a bacterial infection such as helicobacter pylori, a strain of bacteria strongly associated with an increased risk of stomach ulcers[2]. The tests offer a unique insight into your gut health and how it may be remedied through dietary changes or other interventions. I would advise you always do these faecal tests in conjunction with a functional medicine practitioner who is qualified in interpreting the results.

I do ask people to consider doing one of these tests before they start the *Reset Your Gut* programme. It is not a prerequisite, but it would give you the ability to see what is the state of your gut bacteria before you start and the improvement at the end of the programme.

Note: Some companies are starting to offer not only gut microbiome sequencing but also extracting DNA from customers' stool samples. Both Amy Loughman at Deakin University and Rob Knight of the University of California are cautious. They say these tests have "tremendous potential" and are optimistic that the science will help improve people's health in the future, but "It's a big leap from identifying microbes that are there, to knowing how to manipulate them to improve health" either directly or with drugs[3].

SIBO bacterial test

SIBO is a condition characterised by an overgrowth in bacteria which results in your body excreting a high level of hydrogen and methane. Simple tests which measure the gases you exhale are available online. Too detailed to go into here, but a restricted dietary intake will help redress the balance of the bacterial overgrowth. I am currently developing a *Reset Your Gut* programme for SIBO sufferers, check it out on my website: www.ryghealth.com.

Home tests

Acid reflux

I mentioned earlier in Chapter 10 that acid reflux and heartburn are, counterintuitively, often a result of not enough stomach acid rather than too much. Try swallowing a tablespoonful of lemon juice the next time you have stomach pain. If the pain decreases you have too little; if it gets worse you have too much, so then go to see your doctor.

Candidiasis

A candida overgrowth is a fungal infection (it is found typically in the mouth, gut and skin but can spread to other areas of the body too). This overgrowth can lead to an imbalance in the gut microbiome and can cause symptoms such as bloating, gas, cramps and either diarrhoea or constipation. The overgrowth can be caused by:

- Antibiotics (they decrease the amount of lactobacillus, 'good bacteria')

- Diabetes

- Weak immune system

- Poor eating habits, including a lot of sugary foods

- Hormonal imbalance near your menstrual cycle

- Stress

- Lack of sleep

- Pregnancy

A simple home test for candida in your stomach is as follows:

Pour yourself a fresh glass of water before going to bed. Upon waking, collect some saliva (not mucus) and spit into the glass. Watch what happens over the next 20 minutes and if you see strings hanging down from the saliva, cloudy specs suspended in the water or heavy saliva at the bottom, then you have candida[4].

Kelly Brogan, a prominent psychiatrist in the functional medicine field, recommends testing for thyroid complications, vitamin B12 deficiencies, inflammation markers (CRP), fasting, glucose and vitamin

D[5], in order to treat the causes of mental health and not just mask them. I would advise anyone struggling with a mental health challenge to fully consider the benefits of knowing the results of these; you will then be able to take control and understand the health challenges you have rather than trying to guess the cause of your condition.

I have also added other tests that can be useful, but this is only a guideline to start off your journey to better health. Please see a functional medicine practitioner for a full consultation if you can. As we have seen in Chapter 5, a healthy gut microbe balance is essential to good mental health.

Thyroid function test

Your thyroid is the power house of your body that stores and produces hormones that affect the function of virtually every organ in your body.

This test will tell you how well your thyroid gland and immune system are working and assess whether your brain is able to adequately detect your thyroid hormone level. Many things in our western diet disrupt the thyroid function such as trans fats, artificial ingredients, industrial chemicals, gluten (the body can react to this by producing antibodies which attack thyroid tissue) and caffeine. White sugar and refined flour can also negatively affect the thyroid by disrupting stress hormones and affect the makeup of the gut biome[6].

Thyroid: produces T3 and T4 hormones which control your metabolism. T3 is produced from T4 and is the biologically active form. The levels of T3 and T4 that your thyroid produces are controlled by the hormone called TSH which is made by the pituitary gland in the brain[7].

When? If you feel inexplicably tired and have problems controlling your weight, it is worth considering whether your thyroid is the problem. Hypothyroidism means your thyroid is not active enough and isn't producing enough hormone for your needs. Common symptoms of having an underactive thyroid include weight gain, depression, dull hair, constipation and difficulty concentrating. Hyperthyroidism means the opposite: too much hormone is being produced. This can result in weight loss, anxiety, sleeping issues, diarrhoea, rapid heart rate and vision problems.

How? Your doctor can do a blood test for thyroid function by testing the levels of T3, T4 and TSH. Most labs will test for levels of the 'free' form of the hormone which is the biologically active form.

Results: Conventionally, an underactive thyroid can be treated by supplementing synthetic versions of the hormones to raise your thyroxine levels. This is usually a lifelong treatment. An overactive thyroid can be treated with medication to stop your thyroid producing so much hormone.

However, thyroid disorders are usually autoimmune – meaning your body's immune system incorrectly sees the thyroid cells as 'invaders' and tries to destroy them. This can be checked by your doctor using an antibody panel[8]. Dr Mariette Grant, a functional medic practising at www.myspecialistgp.co.uk, identified one patient with very low T3 and T4 despite being on medication to treat it. She also looked at the patient's hormone and vitamin D levels and found they were both low. (Grant explains that, historically, doctors rarely bother treating the autoimmune aspect of the condition, but as a functional medic she was keen to understand how this could happen.)

The patient was also menopausal and, as Dr Grant said: "When you lose your female hormones, oestrogen and progesterone, which are very anti-inflammatory, autoimmune conditions can flare up. Vitamin D is also important to regulate your immunity and it has been shown recently that low vitamin D on its own can cause high blood pressure."

She started prescribing the patient bioidentical hormones and vitamin D supplementations and advised her to stop eating anything which contained gluten. With this approach the patient's thyroid levels stabilised and her blood pressure dropped. This is functional medicine at its best.

Blood tests

We have discussed some key vitamins and minerals needed to keep us all in tip top condition such as iron, zinc and magnesium (to name just a few). It is possible to order detailed blood tests to establish your levels of these from labs like Invivo Clinical and Genova.

Vitamin B12 (folate) and other B vitamins

B12 is critical to brain health and it is an amazing antidepressant[9] keeping our red blood cells, nerve cells and brains functioning properly. B12 deficiency is linked to deep depression, paranoia and memory loss[10].

Dr Brogan likes to see her patients above 600pg/ml and would want to complement the blood level test for B12 with testing for homocysteine levels – an inflammatory protein that is metabolised by B12. A higher level homocysteine will indicate low levels of B12. When she sees low levels, she recommends B12 to decrease the inflammation that could be directly impacting the brain. High levels of homocysteine are a risk factor for a number of diseases including cardiovascular disease and neuropsychiatric illness[11].

Methylation is a biochemical process that is required by many of your body's systems (it controls homocysteine, recycles molecules needed for detoxification, and keeps inflammation under control). Methylation needs folate, B2, B6, B12 and betaine to work effectively, and is impacted amongst other things by poor diet, especially a lack of green vegetables, fruit and foods with naturally occurring B vitamins. A comprehensive blood test will give an indication of your levels.

Vitamin D

Vitamin D is important for absorption of key elements (including calcium and magnesium) and for our immune response. Many factors influence our bodies' abilities to absorb vitamin D. The most extreme outcome of vitamin D deficiency is rickets which results in soft bones. Increasingly recognised risk outcomes of more moderate vitamin D deficiency include cognitive impairment and poor muscular coordination[12]. If you have a vitamin D deficiency you can supplement your diet. Although the primary source of vitamin D is sunlight, it can also be found in food such as fatty fish. Many foods are also fortified with vitamin D.

Further tests recommended by Dr Brogan you might want to consider:

Fasting insulin and haemoglobin A1C

Fasting insulin will indicate how the pancreas is working when you are fasting and the A1C test will give an average of your blood sugar levels over the past 90 days. Recently, glucose monitoring devices for adults with diabetes are allowing millions of people to track their blood sugar levels without having to prick their fingers.

C-reactive protein test (CRP test)

This test, introduced in Chapter 6, can be used to assess the presence of infection or inflammation in your body by measuring the levels of C-reactive protein (CRP) circulating in your blood.

The production of CRP, exclusively occurring in the liver, typically increases in response to inflammation (often due to infection) and can be detected in the blood. High levels of CRP may suggest a patient is suffering from an autoimmune disease or an inflammatory condition. It is used to check for infection after surgery, and to evaluate the effectiveness of treatment in chronic illnesses like lupus and rheumatoid arthritis.

Blood glucose

Unstable blood sugar levels can manifest itself in all sorts of symptoms from panic attacks to fatigue and, of course, as diabetes. There is a blood glucose test available that can screen for diabetes – a condition that arises when your body's systems for maintaining a stable blood sugar level are not working correctly.

One in ten people with the condition have type 1 diabetes, an autoimmune condition where the body is unable to produce insulin (the hormone that transports glucose to the cells). Type 2 diabetes, on the other hand, occurs when insulin is either produced in insufficient quantities or is not properly responded to by the cells in the body. While type 1 is genetic, type 2 diabetes can be determined by lifestyle factors (although there is a genetic component too, of course) and is most common in overweight and obese people. Symptoms include feeling thirsty and tired, weight loss, blurred vision and recurrent candidiasis (thrush). You can assess your risk yourself by visiting the Diabetes UK website (diabetes.org.uk), but if you are genuinely concerned, a trip to the doctor should be your first port of call.

Why? Diabetes is a serious condition that affects over 4 million people in the UK and costs the NHS billions of pounds a year. Research by Public Health England revealed that a quarter of people who have diabetes in England don't even realise they have the life-threatening condition[13]. Going undiagnosed can be dangerous as diabetes can lead to a whole host of health problems, including an increased risk of heart disease and stroke, nerve damage, vision loss and blindness, kidney problems, miscarriage and stillbirth. Dr Grant states that: "Insulin resistance is now believed to be connected to conditions like polycystic ovaries and hormonal imbalances and this can be triggered by having too much sugar and can be unfavourable to the balance of the gut bacteria as well."

How? You will be asked for a urine sample by your doctor. They will test your sample for the presence of sugar in the urine, which is typically not present in healthy samples. If your urine test is positive, you will be given a blood test to determine your sensitivity to glucose – a glucose tolerance test. This blood test requires that you fast beforehand. You will be asked to drink a glucose-containing solution after giving your first sample before being retested two hours later. Alternatively, you may instead be given a glycated haemoglobin test. This test does not require a fasting period. For more information, see the www.nhs.uk website.

Cortisol test

This is a test for adrenal function via giving saliva four times per day. Dr Grant had a patient who was in her mid-thirties looking to conceive her third child. She had regular menstrual cycles, so she checked her thyroid and adrenal function. The patient's thyroid levels were good, but her cortisol was low with no normal fluctuations during the day (see CAR in Chapter 4). Interestingly, the patient did not view her lifestyle as particularly stressful but was advised to reduce her stress levels with exercise and meditation nonetheless. It seemed to do the trick: she is now pregnant with her third child.

Dr Grant stresses that it is a multi-pronged approach that works best. Take another example: a male patient came in asking for a specific drug, well known for increasing concentration and energy levels. She convinced him initially to test his testosterone levels, which turned out to be low. However, he did not improve even when his levels were optimised so she then moved on to checking his thyroid and found he was iodine deficient. The combination of the testosterone and a very low dose iodine supplement, while also increasing the iodine in his diet, did the trick.

Hormones

We know all too well how our hormones affect our mood and sense of wellbeing, but how do they work and why do we need them?

Dr Grant is keen to raise awareness of how fundamental good hormonal balance is to your health and the effect of oral contraception on women's mental health. When the body metabolises oral contraceptive hormones, it causes them to bind to cortisol – a hormone that influences our state of alertness and stress. Grant says doctors need to be aware of this, as prescribing oral contraceptives can therefore affect the way we cope with the daily ups and downs of life. In effect, the pill can block your coping abilities and may even result in doctors then prescribing you antidepressants. Detoxification of the oestrogen is key, and this is done via what you eat. Dr Grant recommends the *Reset Your Gut* programme when she suspects patients are not eating enough fibre to detoxify hormones. So, let's look at each hormone in detail.

Oestrogen

Produced by the ovaries, oestrogen is responsible for a girl's development in puberty and the working of the menstrual cycle.

It also protects the heart by inhibiting plaque in the arteries, and it keeps our bones strong, reducing the risk of osteoporosis[14]. Researchers in Germany have found that women with higher oestrogen levels look younger as it increases collagen in skin[15].

So far, so good. During the menopause, however, the ovaries stop releasing oestrogen (a small amount is still produced from subcutaneous fat[16]). Therefore, it isn't healthy for menopausal women to be too thin. The loss of oestrogen can result in symptoms like vaginal dryness and recurrent urinary tract infections[17]. Women now have a life expectancy of 83, so could be living without oestrogen for 30 years, with all that seems to entail (stomach fat, increased headaches, osteoporosis etc). Plant oestrogen supplements or bio identical (they can also include testosterone, progesterone and DHEA) can have a balancing effect on the body and reduce the impact of the menopause. It is also known that oestrogen can provide some protection against heart disease – the leading cause of death in women after the menopause. In addition, the post-menopausal use of oestrogen seems to delay and decrease the risk of Alzheimer's disease[18].

We supplement if we have low thyroid, why not other hormones? Fortunately, there are a growing number of functional health practitioners specialising in this area – seek them out.

Progesterone

This hormone prepares the body for pregnancy. It supports regular menstrual bleeding, but if your levels are too low it might result in heavy or irregular menstrual bleeding[19], miscarriage[20] or early birth[21]. Progesterone also helps to protect us from endometrial and breast cancer[22].

Oxytocin

Known as the 'love hormone', oxytocin can also promote pleasure and rises in the body during orgasm. This magical chemical reduces stress, induces self-esteem and helps us to calm and bond with our babies. It may even be passed on to them through breastfeeding[23].

And if that wasn't good enough, you can get your fix anywhere. Just hugging someone or being around nature will prompt your brain to start releasing oxytocin.

Testosterone

Considered the most important hormone for men, testosterone is responsible for male development during puberty, and helps to maintain sex drive, sperm production, muscle strength and bone density. Levels of testosterone in men decline very gradually as they get older.

Low testosterone can result in erectile dysfunction, reduced libido and sperm count, and increased propensity to bone damage. Testosterone replacement therapy is available in injections, patches and gels, but there can be side effects[24]. Consider going to a functional health practitioner and having your blood testosterone levels tested, then supplement with natural plant-based testosterone if this is needed.

Genetic testing

Epigenetics is the study of how environmental influences can alter expression of our genes rather than the actual genes themselves and is a fast-growing area of medicine. It is exciting and could, perhaps, pave the way for a new era of personalised medicine. However, the field is still in its infancy, having come about as recently as 2003 with the publication of the first draft of the human genome. There is still so much that remains unknown about the manner in which environment affects our genes. Please make sure you do the tests in conjunction with a qualified genetic counsellor, as it is essential you receive clinical confirmation of the best approach if you receive a positive result. See my website www.maphealthsolutions for a qualified nutritionist who specialises in interpreting epigenetic tests.

What will you find out?

You may think you have a genetic susceptibility to a certain condition or you might just suspect that you are vulnerable to an illness that has hounded your family for generations. Either way, today's modern tests can give you a clearer idea of whether you have inherited a rogue gene or not.

So, what can you do if you have a genetic predisposition to a condition? It is important to remember that predisposition is not the same as a confirmed diagnosis – your genes do not decide your fate!

The idea that having a faulty gene automatically causes a specific condition is just not true. Epigenetics looks at changes in gene expression that do not involve the underlying DNA but do affect how our cells read the genes. Epigenetic change is a regular and normal occurrence and is influenced by several factors such as the state of our gut microbiome, our age, environmental factors and our lifestyle. While some may claim no preventative measures can be taken if you have a specific gene associated with a condition, this is not the case in the slightest. We can influence our genes by paying attention to what will affect them epigenetically.

Now for some scientific detail! Levels of serotonin, the so-called 'happy hormone', are controlled by the action of a gene called SERT (serotonin transporter). There are two common variations in this gene, termed short ('s') and long ('l'). The 's' variant results in a functional reduction of SERT [25]. Studies have indicated that people with the 's' variant are more prone to depression under stressful conditions than those with the 'l' variant[26,27].

In 2004, Joan Kaufman studied depression in maltreated children who received different levels of social support[28]. Unsurprisingly, children with the 's' variant and no positive support network had the highest levels of depression. Encouragingly though, children with the 's' variant who received positive social support had a reduced risk of depression. This shows us that even if you carry a genetic variant associated with an adverse risk, it is possible to modify the outcome!

Nutrigenomics is a branch of epigenetics that enables us to understand the unique interaction between your nutrition and your genes, especially in relation to taking preventative action to avoid chronic disease. This knowledge can empower you to better control your own health outcomes. There is growing recognition of the vital role of nutrition in disease prevention, and an increasing acceptance of the role that many genes play in disease risk.

The nutrigenomics testing market has become quite crowded in recent years, as cloud-based reporting, lower cost technologies and open access journals have all contributed to lowering the barrier to entry to prospective participants.

Simultaneously, there has been an explosion in the awareness of the public about these tests, and a concomitant desire to access the information they provide. One needs to be selective about choosing a partner in this space, as while all the participants might lay claim to be the 'experts', few of them genuinely are.

I use the DNALIFE tests from Nordic Laboratories, they provide very user-friendly reports on the genetics surrounding your health, diet, sport and hormones. These are followed by a consultation with a nutritional consultant who will suggest the best way forward for you to deal with your results. So aside from disease risk, genetic testing can also give us an insight into what is likely to work for each of us – in relation to sport and nutritional requirements. Another company, myDHAhealth, also produces a personalised dietary and lifestyle plan providing you with key nutrients needed for healthy living and ageing based on a DNA test and a series of questionnaires.

Using both Nordic Labs and 23andMe, I personally have tested positive for the APOE gene that indicates I am at a higher risk of getting Alzheimer's. Do I worry about a life in my old age where I no longer know my loved ones? No, I am pleased to know the risk and feel empowered to follow the Bredesen Protocol developed by Dr Dale Bredesen mentioned in Chapter 12. Knowledge is power. For example, individuals with a particular variant in their genes that mean they have an increased risk of type 2 diabetes[29] can then make more appropriate lifestyle choices.

However, these tests can be expensive, and I think that living healthily is great for prevention of a myriad of health issues.

A frequently mentioned genetic variation mentioned in the media at the moment is the MTHFR gene, which affects the production of the MTHFR enzyme that may indicate you need more of the B group vitamins to support methylation (mentioned earlier). The good news is that you can also support methylation by eating nutrient-dense foods, especially dark green vegetables like kale, watercress and spinach. Eggs, meat, fish and liver are all rich in B6 and B12 and some plant-based foods like avocado, sunflower seeds and pistachios contain B6.

However, as mentioned before, if you are vegan vitamin B12 really needs to be supplemented as stated on the Vegan Society website: "B12 is the only vitamin that is not recognised as being reliably supplied from a varied wholefood, plant-based diet with plenty of fruit and vegetables, together with exposure to the sun" (see advice on www.ryghealth.com).

I repeat it is important to remember that many factors influence a given trait and these tests should be explained by a qualified person to ensure that the genetic test is interpreted correctly[30].

Food intolerance

Food intolerance refers to an inability to digest certain foods properly[31]. Symptoms such as stomach pain, bloating and gas after consuming certain food can indicate that you have a food intolerance. In the UK, it is estimated that 1-2% of adults and 5-8% of children have a food allergy (about 2 million people), but this figure does not include those who are affected by mild food reactions to milk, wheat, sugar, seafood, alcohol, nuts, soya and eggs. So the number of people living with food allergy and/or food intolerance is considerably more[32]. They often play a part in triggering gut problems, which is why, in my *Reset Your Gut* programme, we remove inflammatory foods to allow the gut to rebalance its microbiome.

A nutritionist can offer food allergy testing, but the tests are not approved by some in the mainstream medical profession and, in some cases, dismissed as bad science[33]. Personally, I would take a middle ground and recognise that whilst some tests offered cannot be scientifically validated, this also does not prove that food has not been the cause. Common sense should prevail and removing foods, suspected of being inflammatory, as an initial step, and then reintroducing gradually seems a good approach.

In response to an accusation that food intolerance testing was 'bad medicine', Michelle Berriedale-Johnson of Food Matters stated: "A significant amount of people suffer from either chronic or intermittent, indeterminate, 'idiopathic' ill health problems (irritable bowel syndrome, fatigue, joint pains, chronic headache, low-level depression etc.)… and in the vast majority of these cases, their GPs can provide them with neither an explanation nor a treatment for their conditions. This means patients suffer in silence (or clog up their GPs' waiting lists) whilst others seek an answer elsewhere – some experiment with homeopathy, or yoga, or traditional Chinese medicine."

Whilst there aren't specific diagnostic tests for most food intolerances, lactose and fructose are an exception.

Lactose intolerance

Lactose is a type of sugar found mainly in milk and dairy products, and if you're unable to digest it or are intolerant, symptoms can include bloating, stomach cramps, diarrhoea and constipation. There are two ways of definitively testing for lactose intolerance. One is via a blood test taken after you have drunk a lactose solution. If your glucose levels are low this indicates an intolerance as the body is unable to convert the lactose into glucose.

Another way of identifying intolerance is the hydrogen breath test. In this test, you'll be asked to fast for eight to 12 hours before blowing into a bag. You will then be given a lactose solution and your breath will be tested every 15 minutes for levels of hydrogen. If these are high, this will indicate a lactose intolerance as it can cause the bacteria in the colon to produce more hydrogen.

Fructose malabsorption

The hydrogen breath test can also be used for fructose malabsorption. Fructose is a sugar found in fresh fruit and vegetables, honey and many processed foods. Some people struggle to absorb fructose in the small intestine which means it travels on to the colon undigested, reacting with bacteria to cause bloating, stomach cramps and other digestive problems.

Summing up

- Your genetics are not your destiny, you can switch your genes on and off with your lifestyle

- It's not just *your* genes that affect your health but also the genes in your microbiome

- Consider obtaining a gut bacteria profile to design a personalised diet plan

Notes:

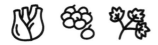

CHAPTER 12

Keep your marbles!

G etting older is something many of us dread, but advancing age doesn't necessarily mean a reduced quality of life, and it is not a given that your memory or mental faculties will diminish with age. In this chapter, we will look at how you can protect yourself from forgetfulness, brain fog and dementia by making changes now that will help you embrace every new decade in the future.

Researchers at the University of California have discovered, by following the lives of 4,000 Italians, that the chances of dying in your 80s and 90s of heart disease, dementia, stroke, cancer and pneumonia are high. But if you survive this, your odds of dying level out after the age of 105 for the next five years and you are more likely to reach 110!

There is an argument that says that to live life to the full, you need to eat, drink and be merry – I respect this choice. I am passionate about the quality of that life, I want to live to the full without any mental or physical health challenges for as long as possible. Put another way: when a car crashes into a brick wall, it is not the brick wall that caused the damage, it's the driving!

So, this chapter is all about driving away from that wall and embracing the ageing process by learning to treat your body well.

Cognitive decline

Have you ever got to the bottom of a page and had to start again from the top, with no recollection of what you've just read? Perhaps you can no longer recall phone numbers that you once knew off by heart, or are becoming increasingly forgetful and finding it difficult to complete tasks that you could once do with ease. According to Age Concern UK, mild cognitive impairment affects between 5% and 20% of people over the age of 65, although often not significantly enough to affect their ability to live independently[1]. However, regardless of its severity, the regular 'senior moments' associated with such cognitive decline can be both debilitating and embarrassing.

Alzheimer's and other forms of dementia

The Alzheimer's Society states there are currently 850,000 people living with dementia in the UK with this set to rise to over 1 million by 2025, and 2 million by 2051. The WHO estimates that 47 million people worldwide are living with some sort of dementia and predict that this will rise to around 75 million by 2030 and 132 million by 2050.

The most common type of dementia is Alzheimer's disease, a neurodegenerative condition responsible for two out of three cases of significant cognitive decline. Symptoms typically begin with forgetfulness and confusion, but can escalate to dramatic mood swings, inability to follow instructions and language disturbances as the disease progresses. Alzheimer's is initially a physical disease that affects the brain, reducing the effectiveness of neuronal connections, eventually leading to the permanent loss of brain tissue. This results in such severe cognitive impairment that most sufferers become completely incapacitated, unable to recognise the faces of loved ones or to carry out the very simplest of tasks.

Unless a cure or a way to avoid dementia is found, it is predicted that up to 2 million people in the UK will have dementia by 2051. The cost of this illness, in its various forms, currently stands at £26bn a year in the UK alone, which equates to an annual bill of around £31,000 per patient per year. The impact of dementia is financial as well as physical, psychological and emotional[2].

Reversal of cognitive decline

It is generally accepted that losing your cognitive faculties is an inevitable part of growing older, but it doesn't have to be. There are many changes you can make to prevent cognitive decline from shaping your later years[2].

My father, a doctor who finished his career at the top of the occupational medicine field, sadly died of Alzheimer's in 2010. The only treatment available for him at the time was drugs. Thankfully, while there is still no cure for dementia, there is now the possibility of positive intervention without drugs.

I first became aware of this approach when listening to Dr Mary Newport speak at the Awakening from Alzheimer's conference in 2016. She is a doctor who specialises in the treatment of premature babies. She used MCT oil to help them grow faster, as this oil is easily absorbed by the body and can be used directly by the brain as an energy source (bypassing the glucose route to supply the brain with energy). Dr Newport's husband developed Alzheimer's and she described a "perfect storm" where her previous knowledge collided with her life experience.

Researchers have found there is often an insulin deficiency and resistance in people who die of Alzheimer's and it is known as the '3rd diabetes'. She decided to give her husband MCT oil (a saturated fat found in coconut oil) in every form possible, thereby bypassing the need for insulin to be present to supply his brain with glucose. It was remarkable: his symptoms reversed. At the time it was controversial, as saturated fat was seen by many in the medical community as the reason for heart disease. But Dr Newport's husband, and subsequently patients of hers, used this approach and managed to "stop Alzheimer's in its tracks".

Of course, some of the drug companies dismissed the effects as anecdotal, and doctors needed more research to be confident in encouraging their patients to stop taking the drugs they had been taught to prescribe at medical school. Thankfully, this has happened.

A recent, ground-breaking study by Dr Dale Bredesen, an international expert in degenerative diseases, revealed that a comprehensive therapeutic regime can improve cognitive function. He employed a combination of a behavioural approach and functional medicine to treat ten patients with early stage Alzheimer's disease. The programmes included a low-carb, gluten-free diet, rich in fruit, vegetables, wild fish, B12 and other vitamin mineral supplementation, probiotics and coconut oil like Dr Mary Newport also used in her regime.

It includes a regular fasting programme, various de-stressing interventions, including meditation and yoga, plus melatonin, the sleep hormone, to ensure good sleep. He also incorporated coffee concentrate into the protocol, as this has been shown to increase the production of Brain Derived Neurotrophic Factors (BDNF) – a hormone that promotes the growth of new brain cells. See Chapter 7 on other benefits of coffee.

After six months, nine out of the ten participants experienced a substantial improvement in cognitive function, to the extent that six of the volunteers were able to return to their jobs, having given up work when their symptoms first began[3,4]. This is remarkable stuff, and with no drug taken! Drug companies are trialling vaccines they hope will reverse dementia, but I would suggest that the lifestyle changes and protocol detailed above is a more sustainable option.

In 2018, Dr Bredesen presented to the World Bank on the economics of Alzheimer's disease, addressing the fact that billions of dollars have been invested in studies trying to find a magic 'drug bullet' to prevent the physical changes associated with the development of Alzheimer's (eg the accumulation of a sticky protein called beta-amyloid). Unfortunately, all have failed. In fact, recent practice guidelines[5] for neurologists based on studies of the medications available indicated that clinicians should inform patients about the lack of evidence supporting the effectiveness of these drug treatments and suggest lifestyle alterations (such as regular exercise[6]) instead. I don't imagine that's something the drug companies would like to hear!

It is becoming more and more obvious that obesity and ageing is linked to Alzheimer's markers in the brain[7]. So, if you feel you need to implement some positive lifestyle changes, consider signing up for the *Reset Your Gut* programme, designed to help you turn your attitude to health around while remaining simple, accessible and affordable.

In Chapter 6 I discussed the effect inflammation can have on cognitive decline. Research by Dr Mary Morris also suggests that inflammation is involved with the development of Alzheimer's disease. He demonstrated that there was a decreased risk of developing dementia if you had a high level of DHA – the all-important omega-3[8]. Omega-3 is thought to interact with, and turn on, the gene responsible for manufacturing BDNF and thus promoting the growth of new brain cells.

Dr Dale Bredesen has also shown that DHA can assist your body in dealing with excess inflammation[9,10], another factor associated with the development of Alzheimer's. Dr Bredesen has very specific advice when it comes to oil choice, suggesting that we focus on consuming oils that are high in omega-3 and not omega-6 (as this is involved in increasing inflammation). Such oils are found in products such as olives and avocados.

An integrative approach

Studies like Dr Bredesen's are very encouraging and they support the approach that early intervention can reverse the symptoms of cognitive decline. I have seen first-hand that paying attention to your microbiome promotes communication between our two brains – the one in our head and the one in our gut. I have worked with a patient who complained of low mood, irritability and decreasing concentration. I encouraged him to have a blood and stool test, which showed he was lacking in certain vitamins and minerals and his gut was not in balance (he had a dysbiosis, an excess of opportunistic bacteria).

Then I started him on the *Reset Your Gut* programme. We removed inflammatory foods, gave him stomach enzymes, increased his pre- and probiotic intake and helped him restore his gut lining. I used CBT and EFT as part of his specialised intervention plan. The result was remarkable: he felt so different. His brain was able to function optimally, and it appeared by healing his gut dysbiosis, his mental state improved. I respect that scientists will say this is purely anecdotal, but this integrative approach seemed to be successful in this case.

What can you do?

Food for your brain

At any age, but particularly as we get older, food can exert a hugely positive influence on brain function. Research has revealed that people who regularly eat fish[11], fruit, vegetables and little dairy or red meat, experience a much slower rate of memory loss than their less diet-conscious counterparts. Excess alcohol, red meat, salt, sugar and an excess of saturated fats can all have a detrimental effect on brain health[12]. In line with Chapter 2, where we advised eating saturated fats in lower amounts, it has been demonstrated that people who eat a higher amount of saturated fat over a six-year period had a higher risk of developing Alzheimer's disease[13].

Mediterranean diet

No fewer than 13 different studies have revealed that a Mediterranean diet can be linked to slowing the rate of cognitive decline, and slower onset of age-related conditions such as Alzheimer's disease[14] and macular degeneration[15]. There is also evidence to suggest that a Mediterranean diet helps to reduce inflammation and lower cholesterol, both of which have been linked to an increased risk of dementia, memory loss and other cognitive problems[16].

With that in mind, it's important to load up on berries, nuts, olive oil and seafood to keep your brain firing well into old age[17]. The Global Council on Brain Health says the same thing and recommends eating plenty of green leafy vegetables and consuming plenty of omega-3 rich foods to help protect you from dementia.

With these studies in mind, the *Rest Your Gut* programme has specific vegetarian and/or vegan options available as well as meat options with lots of vegetables included.

Vitamin D

A large observational study published in *Neurology* suggests that people with very low levels of vitamin D in their blood are more than twice as likely as those with normal vitamin D levels to develop Alzheimer's disease or other types of dementia (though more research is needed to show cause and effect). However, as vitamin D is vital to bone metabolism, calcium absorption and other metabolic processes in the body, and some studies suggest that vitamin D may be involved in a variety of processes related to cognition, it can do no harm to get outside every day[18].

Dr Dean Sherzai and Dr Ayesha Sherzai, co-authors of *The Alzheimer's Solution*, recommend these foods to protect your brain from decline[19]:

- Avocado

- Beans

- Blueberries

- Sweet potatoes

- Extra virgin olive oil

- Linseeds

- Leafy green vegetables

- Nuts

- Spices (especially turmeric, cinnamon, saffron)

- Tea (green tea, mint, lemon balm)

- Wholegrains

Foods to avoid:

- Trans fats (crisps, biscuits, margarine)

- Processed meat (bacon, sausages, smoked hams)

- Sugar (pastries, sweets, biscuits, cakes)

- Sugary drinks

- Excessive alcohol

Insulin resistance

Insulin resistance occurs when your body cells fail to respond normally to insulin, leading to a build-up of glucose in the bloodstream. This, in turn, can lead to serious health conditions, such as type 2 diabetes.

However, it probably won't surprise you to know that insulin resistance has also been linked to dementia and Alzheimer's disease; as stated earlier, it is also known as the '3rd diabetes'. A study by the University of Tel Aviv revealed that people who are insulin resistant have a higher risk of poor cognitive performance and cognitive decline. The precise mechanisms underpinning this are unclear, although damage to blood vessels by high glucose levels or the direct effects of a lack of insulin on the brain have been proposed as potential contributors[20]. Either way, there appears to be a link between insulin resistance and dementia.

Prevention

So, if you want to reduce your chances of developing dementia or Alzheimer's, the above evidence suggests you should also be safeguarding yourself from insulin resistance and diabetes. Being obese or overweight, eating a diet high in carbs and sugar, not exercising enough, chronic stress and the long-term use of steroids are all risk factors for insulin resistance and are thus best avoided if you wish to keep your brain firing on all cylinders[21]. Need help avoiding insulin resistance? Yes, you guessed it: the *Reset Your Gut* programme could be for you!

Restorative sleep

There is a definite link between poor sleep and reduced cognitive ability. Sleep problems have been found to raise levels of certain proteins in the brain tissue associated with Alzheimer's. These deposits accumulate in the brain every day, and your brain will naturally sweep them away when you are asleep. A study by Maiken Nedergaard and her colleagues at the University of Rochester demonstrated how the amyloid beta component of these protein plaques (the component primarily linked to Alzheimer's) is cleared twice as quickly in mice that are asleep compared to ones that are awake [22]. If sleep is disturbed, however, the cleansing process can't happen as effectively. Although no equivalent experiment has been carried out on humans, it has been suggested that our waste disposal system may work in a similar way.

Sleeping position

Your sleeping position can also affect the efficiency of the brain's self-cleansing process. In another test by the same group at the University of Rochester, it was revealed that mice that slept on their sides experienced more effective brain cleansing than mice that slept on their backs[23].

How many hours?

The authors of *The Alzheimer's Solution* agree that one of our biggest defences against dementia is sleep. They state that getting between seven and eight hours of good quality shut-eye every night helps to keep your brain healthy. Not only does it give you time to clear out unwanted toxins, but also reduces inflammation, regenerates the neurons and makes you less likely to crave the high-sugar foods you are automatically drawn to when you are tired.

Earlier, I suggest that people should be having at least seven hours sleep a night; however, another study by Boston University found that older people who routinely have more than nine hours a night double their risk of developing dementia. It is not yet known why this is, but it is likely that the need for a lie-in is in fact an early sign rather than a cause of dementia[24].

Keep moving

Being active is at the heart of a healthy lifestyle at any age, but becomes increasingly important as you start to get older. In fact, American researchers claim that exercising regularly can cut your risk of developing Alzheimer's disease in half. So why is this?

Although the precise mechanisms remain unclear, researchers at the University of Pittsburgh have suggested that this may be due to the effect of exercise on regions of the brain that are typically found to deteriorate as Alzheimer's progresses. More specifically, the size of the hippocampus and the prefrontal cortex (parts of the brain involved in memory formation and complex thinking) has been found to correlate with frequency of exercise and fitness levels. This suggests that exercise can actually help your brain to grow, warding off the threat of dementia[25].

How much and what?

Even if you're a born couch potato. don't despair! Keeping active doesn't necessarily mean endless gym sessions.

Dr Kirk Erikson, the researcher in charge of the above Pittsburgh study, got 100 men and women aged 60 to 80 to walk for about 40 minutes, three times a week, for a year. Remarkably, at the end of the study year, their hippocampi had grown by an average of 2%. This might not sound a lot, but when we consider that older adults typically display a 1-2% decrease in hippocampal volume each year, a 2% increase is huge! In addition to measurable brain growth, the participants also showed improvements in performance on memory tests compared to before the study[26].

I love to dance and have recently qualified as a DDMIX instructor – a dance fitness programme created by the famous ballerina Dame Darcey Bussell DBE – with the intention of teaching a weekly class in a local nursing home. A study by the Centre for Neurodegenerative Diseases in Magdeburg, Germany, has shown (to my delight) that out of two types of exercise done for 90 minutes (dancing and endurance/strength/flexibility training) dance has the most profound effect[27]. It was found that dance exercise was associated with greater increase in the hippocampus area of the brain concerned with memory, learning and emotion.

So, get up and makes some moves to your favourite beat!

Body and mind

According to Alzheimer's Research UK, many of the risk factors associated with cardiovascular disease (eg stroke and heart disease) can also contribute to the development of dementia. This is especially true in the case of vascular dementia, which is caused by reduced blood supply to the brain due to vessel damage[28]. With this in mind, it makes sense that looking after your body will inevitably have a positive effect on your brain[29].

Dynamic ageing

This is the idea that we can all take a proactive approach towards our health and wellbeing and, in doing so, can slow the ageing process.

By exercising regularly, socialising and really engaging with the world around you, you have a far better chance of staying mobile, healthy and energetic for as long as possible. At the forefront of this health philosophy is 'biomechanistic' author Katy Bowman. Below are some of her suggestions for increasing strength and mobility[30]:

- Stretch: To keep your body as supple as possible.

- Embrace nature: Try to exercise in green (forests, woods, parks) and blue (beach, riverside) spaces as often as you can. Being out in the open air on varied surfaces is restorative and improves balance.

- Exercise with friends: Instead of meeting up for a coffee, why not arrange to go for a walk instead? It will make your workout more fun and uplifting.

- Meditation: Researchers at the University of California have found that people who meditate for up to an hour a day have better cognitive abilities than those who mediate less or not at all. Furthermore, immediately after an intensive meditation retreat, participants showed "improvements in attention, general psychological wellbeing and a better ability to cope with stress. The benefits continued after the retreat especially for those who continued meditating" [31]. I am sure this is only one way of increasing cognitive abilities and it will not suit everyone to dedicate an hour a day to mediation, so aim for ten minutes initially and see how you go.

Mindset – 'we become what we think about'

As we have already seen in this book, our outlook not only contributes to our susceptibility to mental health problems but can also affect our physical state. This doesn't change as we get older and is worth paying attention to.

Depression

A comprehensive study undertaken recently by the University of Pittsburgh's School of Medicine concluded that older people with late-onset depression were 65% more likely to develop Alzheimer's disease and 152% more at risk of ending up with vascular dementia. The mechanism behind the link is still not clear, but the scientists involved in this study have suggested that depression-associated changes in the brain may increase subjects' vulnerability to developing dementia[32]. While this may sound scary to anyone prone to depression, the good news is that depression can be treated effectively through talking therapies, lifestyle changes and medication. The key, as always, is to be proactive about your health and to get help when you need it. Doing the RYG programme would be a great start.

Rumination

We've all been there: lying wide awake at 3am, desperately worrying about a problem. Unpleasant though it is, there's nothing unusual about the occasional sleepless night. In fact, reflection is a perfectly normal part of problem solving! However, when worrying spills over into rumination – the habit of rehashing worries or regrets over and over again in our minds – it can put our bodies under chronic stress. This can lead to an elevated heart rate, increased blood pressure and a higher risk of anxiety and depression[33]. On top of this, anxiety and depression have actually been linked to shortened telomeres (the part of the chromosome responsible for ageing) so getting stressed can, quite literally, speed up ageing[34].

Next time you find yourself getting het up or overwhelmed by a problem, take a step back and evaluate your approach before diving in at the deep end and stressing yourself out. As the saying goes, you really can worry yourself sick. You may also want to consider doing some CBT therapy available online or with a therapist. For more information, visit my website: www.maphealthsolution.com.

Brain training

Numerous studies have shown that regularly challenging our grey matter through continuous learning and testing can improve our cognitive ability. This trend was set in motion by a recent study from the University of California in which the participants, all aged over 60, were challenged to play specially formulated 'brain training video games' for at least three hours a week. After a month, the volunteers were tested and showed substantial improvements in memory, attention and their ability to multitask[35]. This is great news for all of us, as it suggests that our brains are even more elastic and pliable than we thought. If you challenge yourself regularly to learn something new, your brain will continue to adapt and grow regardless of how old you are.

Use it or lose it

As we have seen, getting older isn't necessarily something to worry about. By making positive changes to your lifestyle now, you have a good chance of staying happy, healthy and on the ball for many years to come. A few key points to remember:

- Try to stick to a diet high in fresh fruit, vegetables, nuts and fat from plant sources

- Aim for seven to eight hours of undisturbed sleep a night

- Exercise, stretch and enjoy being active

- Look on the bright side and keep challenging your brain

- If you're worried about cognitive decline, seek help as soon as possible

- Avoid trans fats, processed meat, refined sugar and excess alcohol

- Maintain a healthy weight

- Consider learning something new – use it or lose it

Notes:

Notes:

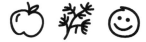

CHAPTER 13

What you can do today for tomorrow

Many of us often find ourselves so busy that we tend to plaster over our health problems rather than making an effort to get to the root of them. Unfortunately, this approach clearly isn't working: the number of prescriptions has doubled in the last decade[1] and more people than ever are suffering from chronic conditions. In a global status report issued by the WHO in 2012, non-communicable diseases (NCDs are chronic diseases that begin to develop long before symptoms appear) were stated to be a "leading cause of death globally". In fact, NCD's were responsible "for 38 million (68%) of the world's 56 million deaths in 2012".

Currently the WHO states that non-communicable diseases (not caused by infection) like heart disease, obesity, cancer, and even psychological disorders like depression, kill three times as many people worldwide (69% of deaths) as infectious diseases (23% of deaths). The rate in western cultures rises to 87% of deaths[2] but this proportion is on the rise in low- to middle-income countries as well. Public health in developing countries is improving and infectious diseases are declining, but chronic diseases are increasing and disproportionately striking younger people. This is being attributed in part to the urbanisation of populations and their exposure to poor nutrition and air pollution[3].

NCDs cannot be passed on; they are a symptom of your body being out of balance, and while drug companies can make money out of masking your symptoms and pay taxes on their profits, there is little incentive for any governments to do anything.

Conventional medical practice attempts to combat this by moving away from bad health through prescription drugs and other reactive treatments. I, however, passionately believe (and this is why I do what I do) that we should instead be moving towards good health. Moving towards good health involves loading the dice in your favour through positive changes in your diet, lifestyle and environment. Setting up these habits in younger years can radically alter your chances of rapid decline later in life. That said, it's never too late to start. The human body is amazingly responsive to being treated well, so, regardless of age, the best time to introduce positive changes is always right now.

After all… if you always do what you have always done you will always get what you have always got!

A local cardiologist describes the experience of her husband who has a genetic predisposition to a wide spectrum of autoimmune diseases like psoriasis, inflammation of the middle layer of the eye, and inflammation of the sacroiliac joint. He was prescribed steroids but had to stop because he started developing cataracts. He was prescribed immunosuppressant drugs and, because of her profession, she was aware of the potential serious side effects and was quite shocked at the strength of the drugs he was having to take.

Her husband heard about anti-inflammatory diets (like my RYG programme) and he set out with determination on his own to reduce his inflammation naturally. He read about probiotics and took these. His regime got rid of his uveitis, and although he has minor recurrences of the other conditions, as soon as he follows an anti-inflammatory diet he gets his health back under control. This is a brilliant example of how acting today enabled him to manage a genetic predisposition by balancing his microbiome and reducing the inflammatory load in his body.

Recently, I was asked to work with a friend's mother who, in her seventies, was showing signs of depression. Interestingly, a recent survey by the Royal Society for Public Heath found that one in four millennials thought it was "normal to be depressed in older age". This is not true and quite a defeatist attitude that needs to be challenged. I worked with the mother and helped her change her diet through the RYG programme; her daughter now says there is no stopping her.

"All the time, I see patients who don't need a pill, they need a change of lifestyle," says Dr Rangan Chatterjee, the pioneering GP who features in the BBC series *Doctor in the House*[4].

Chatterjee believes that by making a few small changes and gaining a greater understanding of how our bodies work, we can become happier and healthier individuals. Being open to new ways of solving health issues, without the use of drugs, is so important to allow the functional medical field to develop in conjunction with what medicine does best: treating acute conditions.

In 2015, after I ruptured my anterior cruciate ligament in a skiing accident, I underwent treatment in which stem cells were extracted from my bone marrow by the innovative and talented surgeon Ali Bajwa and injected into the damaged cartilage in my knee. Fast-forward to now and the cartilage in my damaged knee is as good as new with no sign of damage (I am 56 at the age of writing this). This new area of regenerative medicine is exciting and rapidly expanding, with stem cells now being produced from fat cells as well as extracted from bone marrow[5].

This is precisely the sort of direction the medical field should be progressing in: creating innovative and effective ways at solving health problems, not simply prescribing drugs without looking at the root cause. Functional medicine practitioners are trying to do just that, forging forward on this new frontier and helping people improve their health from the inside out.

In this, I want to share just a few simple facts which will make you feel fitter, not just now but in the future. It will save you doing the research!

Water

When you look in the mirror, it's hard to believe that two-thirds of your body weight is made up of water. The fact is, we simply can't survive without it (or not for long, anyway).

So why exactly is it so important to stay hydrated?

Dehydration

It is recommended that you drink between six and eight glasses of water a day[6]. If you don't drink enough, you risk becoming dehydrated and upsetting the balance of salts and sugars in your body, ultimately affecting the way it functions. Early signs of dehydration include feeling thirsty and dizzy, a headache, a dry mouth and dark-coloured urine. Chronic dehydration can even lead to impaired kidney function[7], constipation and muscle damage.

Interestingly, people often confuse the symptoms of dehydration with those of hunger, so it's probably a good idea to have a glass of water before heading for the fridge or a snack when you're feeling peckish.

Liquid benefits

Water is essential to body function. It plays a vital role in enabling us to maintain a stable body temperature, lubricating our eyes and cushioning our joints. It also protects your spinal cord, aids digestion, and helps flush out toxins.

Other drinks and even foods with a high liquid content, such as soups, celery, tomatoes or melons, can help to keep you hydrated.

How warm or cold?

Researchers claim that ice-cold water hydrates the body more quickly and improves exercise endurance[8] while warm water is thought to boost metabolism and helps to aid digestion. Either way, water is good. Personally, I think a cup of warm water with lemon juice squeezed into it is a great start to the day. Be careful with sparkling water, though. It might taste good, but it contains carbonic acid which could damage your tooth enamel[9]. On the other hand, it makes you feel fuller than the plain stuff, so might mean you eat less. I love carbonated water with lemon juice.

So, gentlemen (and ladies because we care too) listen up as we move seamlessly from water to sex.

The connection between erectile dysfunction and heart disease

A study in Minnesota showed that men who reported erectile dysfunction but no heart disease at the time had a 40 to 50 times higher risk of a heart attack within five to ten years[10]. Furthermore, Dr Hackett wrote in the *British Medical Journal* that erection problems are a warning sign that men are at a significant risk of suffering a heart attack[11]. The NHS states that erectile dysfunction has a wide range of known medical causes, and all risk factors should be assessed as well as considering if the patient has the potential for cardiovascular disease[12].

For erectile function you need adequate pelvic blood flow. The key to opening your arteries and allowing blood to flow anywhere in your body is nitric oxide. The endolethium, the lining in all your arteries (which covers the equivalent of six or seven tennis courts) makes nitric oxide, which dilates blood vessels and is thus essential for maintaining healthy blood pressure and healthy arteries[13]. This discovery that nitric oxide is a signalling molecule in the cardiovascular system won three scientists the Nobel Prize for Medicine in 1998[14].

Nitrates may be found in some food including leafy green vegetables and other colourful veg like beetroot. Our body is capable of converting these nitrates into nitric oxide[15] via the endolethium, which then enables your arteries to dilate[16]. As a result, choosing to eat foods that aid endothelial structure and function (fruits, vegetables, wholegrains, legumes) means you're essentially eating natural Viagra!

Viagra, also known as Sildenafil, was originally developed as a drug for heart disease as it had a favourable effect on arterial dilation. By inhibiting an enzyme known as PDE5, associated with muscle contraction in all smooth muscle including penile tissue, Viagra allows blood vessels to relax, leading to increased blood flow into the penis. While its ability to stimulate an erection is undeniable, it's not without its side effects. Viagra becomes less effective with more use as the body's receptors become used to the drug (known as tolerance), ultimately forcing the user to become even more reliant on it.

If you're wondering how to maintain a healthy endothelium, it is quite simple. Studies have shown that "A Mediterranean Diet Improves Erectile Function"[17]. This is not vegan propaganda, it really does. The study followed men who had a metabolic syndrome (this is the name given to patients with a group of risk factors – high blood pressure, high blood sugar, high triglycerides, low HDL cholesterol, and belly fat – that increases risk of heart disease and diabetes). They ate a predominantly Mediterranean-style diet: rich in vegetables, fruit, lentils, beans, wholegrains and nuts and with very little meat. They found men eating in this way were far less likely to experience erectile dysfunction than men eating a typical western diet, which tends to include much more meat.

Note: The nitrates and other chemicals used in processed meats have shown in observational studies that people who eat processed meat over a long period of time may increase the risk of many chronic diseases, such as heart disease and cancer [18].

A film due to be released in 2018 made by James Cameron called *Game Changers,* with the stated aim of creating a 'seismic shift' in the way we eat and live, followed an interesting experiment in which three fit athletic men were fed a plant-based meal, then a meat-based meal, and then measured how many erections they had at night and how frequent they were[19]. What did the urologist Aaron Spitz doing the experiments find? After a plant-based meal the men had 300 to 500 more frequent erections and were 10-15% harder. This is sensational stuff and at the time of writing the film has not been released so we will have to wait and see!

However, it does make sense that what affects your genitals will affect your heart and brain. A healthy diet means a healthy endothelium, and ultimately improved blood flow around the body.

All good reasons to up your greens, boys! Follow the RYG programme and start healing that endothelium.

Nutrients

"Even women who eat an incredibly balanced, wholesome diet can still miss out on the key nutrients necessary for peak health," says nutritionist Dr Michelle Braude[20], author of *The Food Effect.* According to the CDC, 90% of Americans do not eat five servings of fruit and vegetables a day – the minimum required to get the nutrition you need (especially B6, B12 and folate which are all essential for brain health).

If you really are struggling, my advice would be to go and see a functional medicine nutritionist or a medic with nutritional training and ask for a blood test (see Chapter 11). If that is beyond your pocket, then follow a nutritionally balanced programme such the RYG programme to help you balance your nutrient intake and reboot the way you eat, and you can go online to www.ryghealth.com and download a free booklet which will give you guidelines for rebalancing your gut bacteria.

In the meantime, here are some brief details on things to consider.

Vitamin D

If you live in the northern hemisphere you could be severely lacking in the 'sunshine vitamin' – vitamin D, an essential vitamin for bone growth and development[21]. Vitamin D should be at the top of your list to test for, regardless of age, sex, colour, health as it has been linked to a diverse range of heart disease, diabetes, autoimmune conditions, chronic pain, depression, cancer… the list goes on.

Receptors that respond to vitamin D have been found in every type of human cell and it is thought to play a key role in regulating both the immune and neuromuscular system. It also plays major roles in the life cycle of human cells. I was shocked to discover that my daughter, who eats well and regularly spends time outside, was way below the NHS recommended guideline (80 nmol) for serum vitamin D levels at just 45 nmol. I encouraged her to boost her intake of foods naturally high in vitamin D, such as eggs, but also made sure, during the winter, that she took D3, the form naturally produced by your body in sunshine.

Vitamin D is also associated with leptin resistance – the 'satiety' hormone that tells you when you are full[22]. When your vitamin D level is low, your resistance to leptin results in a loss of satiety and increased food cravings. These cravings will go away when you boost your vitamin D levels via sunshine or supplementation[23].

A blood test for vitamin D is available from the NHS and, in my opinion, this is well worth doing[24]. My local functional medicine doctor, Dr Marietta Grant, recommends that everyone gets themselves tested as she has been shocked by the number of people who are deficient. Once you've established if you are deficient, it's also important to look at the possible reasons why this deficiency has occurred rather than just supplementing randomly (this would be hardly different from prescribing drugs).

For instance, high doses of vitamin D can lead to a vitamin K deficiency[25], and a vitamin D deficiency could be a result of interactions with magnesium[26,27]. Over 300 different processes in your body use magnesium including our Krebs cycle – the body's way of creating energy. Interestingly, a study has shown that vitamin D supplementation was more effective at correcting vitamin D deficiency if taken with magnesium than if taken on its own. It is therefore important to get a balance between them all rather than just taking vitamin D supplements and masking the true cause of the problem.

Of course, another way of boosting your vitamin D levels is to go outside and get it naturally! Be careful, though – it's not advisable to go outside for more than 35 minutes between 10am and 3pm without sun cream (see Chapter 9 for advice on choosing sun creams). Vitamin D is great, sunburn is not!

Whilst the Institute of Medicine Expert Committee in 2010 said that presently they would like to see more evidence for some of these claims, a group of scientists have set up the Vitamin D Council to promote vitamin D deficiency awareness. Either way, we need it, so I would strongly urge you to check your levels.

Iron

Iron is essential for producing red blood cells, which carry oxygen around your body to your organs and tissues. To boost your body's iron levels, eat dark leafy greens and legumes such as lentils and kidney beans[28].

Kelly Brogan MD recommends paying special attention to the following for mood and energy regulation[29]:

B12 as it has proven to be among the most useful, safe and effective treatments for many psychiatric conditions.

Magnesium provides relief from ailments such as PMS, poor thyroid function and depression.

Zinc cannot be stored by our bodies and zinc deficiency is often found concurrent with psychiatric disorders and plays an important role in immune system regulation, sexual health and cellular repair.

Essential fatty acids promote cellular growth, build new brain tissue and protect neural pathways. The brain is 60% fat so consuming adequate amounts of healthy fats, as discussed previously, is crucial to good mental health and reducing inflammation. Eating fat will not make you fat, a high natural fat diet has a natural blood sugar stabilising effect.

These can all be obtained by eating a healthy diet. Use the *Rest Your Gut* programme to start doing this today for a healthy tomorrow.

Fibre

According to research by the NHS, most adults in the UK are eating only 60% of the fibre they need to stay healthy (around 30g per day). In contrast, the Hadza tribe in Tanzania consume up to 150g per day! This particular tribe are featured in Jeff D. Leach's book[30] *Rewild* where he investigated the comparison between a typical American's gut bacteria with those of the Hadza tribe. In one extreme experiment, Leach injected himself with their faeces (details in the book) and began following their diet and found his gut microbial diversity increased dramatically as a result.

Fibre is essential for controlling blood sugar levels, lowering cholesterol, and of course, keeping you regular. High-fibre goods include oats, rye, fruit and all vegetables[28]. Fibre is also an essential source of prebiotics that keeps our microbiome healthy and features heavily in the RYG programme.

Why do something today for tomorrow?

Avani Hurribunce, a maths teacher at my daughter's school, told me how she realised that she needed to start taking action to avoid following her family who all suffered from diabetes. She is fourth generation South African, and her ancestors were Indian, settling as indentured labour in

South Africa from 1860. She and her siblings were brought up on a diet of vegetables and rice, supplemented with meat and fish. Surprisingly, all nine of her mother's siblings, as well as Avani's brothers, have diabetes, or did before they died. She herself was diagnosed with diabetes, despite eating a diet consisting mostly of vegetables (albeit with Chinese noodles and white basmati rice).

Initially, she took drugs, but on reading Dr Chatterjee's book *The 4 Pillar Plan*, in which Chatterjee promotes eating well, sleeping, exercise and relaxing, she decided to tackle her diabetes with these lifestyle changes. She is no longer diabetic, has more energy, has lost weight, is back exercising and determined to show her brothers in South Africa, who laughed at her for trying to reverse her diabetes. They could not have been more wrong! Who knows, maybe she'll teach them to reverse theirs.

Interestingly, her approach included three periods of fasting per week, which is one approach I suggest in the RYG programme.

Fasting

The thought of going without food might not be your idea of fun, but bear with me, various studies have shown that not eating for 12 hours or more can be good for you.

Why bother?

Research has revealed that fasting rests your digestive system, reduces inflammation, and can also lower cholesterol and blood sugar. This is because after about 12 hours the body will run out of glucose reserves[31] and will begin burning fat as a source of energy instead, dissolving many of the harmful toxins stored inside it.

And for those with real willpower, why not fast for longer? A new study from researchers at the University of Southern Carolina proves that going without food for as little as three days can completely rejuvenate the immune system[32].

"When you starve, the system tries to save energy, and one of the things it can do to save energy is to recycle a lot of the immune cells that are not needed, especially those that may be damaged," says Dr Longo, who headed up the research project[33]. This seems a little extreme to me and I only recommend in the RYG programme a a maximum of a 12-hour fasting period.

Prolonged fasting can also reduce the enzyme PKA which is linked to ageing[32]. Yep, you heard right: overeating speeds up ageing and can lead to a shorted lifespan. Researchers are also now examining whether fasting can hinder cancer progression[34].

Fasting is not recommended for pregnant or breastfeeding women, if you have a weakened immune system or a history of eating disorders. If you're unsure, please consult with your doctor before attempting any fasting regime.

Tips for fasting:

- Before the fast, stick to lean proteins, healthy fats and complex carbohydrates to provide your body with enough energy

- Drink plenty of water as you will be missing out on liquids from food

- Avoid tea and coffee as they can dehydrate you

- Skip the intense workout as it will make you hungrier and deplete your glucose reserves, go for a walk instead

- Listen to your body and stop if you feel unwell

- Meditate or practise mindfulness

Sleep

We have already seen the importance of sleep in the context of mental health, inflammation and a healthy microbiome, and you will remember that sleep is boosted by exercise.

It is no wonder that sleep is so important – it takes up a third of our life, after all. Good sleep is crucial for your health. Sleep deprivation can lead to a 'fuzzy head', fatigue and lack of motivation in the short term, and long term it can contribute to weight gain, diabetes, heart disease, stroke and memory loss[35].

Feeling irritable, grumpy and fatigued? Look at your sleeping habits, you might be surprised, and do the RYG programme. My wonderful neighbour Courtnay Brennan has recently done this and she calls me her angel, as having not slept properly for 20 years, she now has amazing sleep, has no afternoon dip and is full of energy.

But what exactly is sleep?

A typical night's sleep consists of several cycles alternating between rapid eye movement (REM) sleep and non-REM sleep. REM sleep is associated with random, rapid, side to side eye movements behind the closed eyelids whilst non-REM sleep is not[36].

Sleep begins with non-REM sleep which consists of three distinct phases: stages 1, 2 and 3, with the associated sleep getting deeper with each stage. For example, stage 1 is the transition phase between being awake and asleep, it is associated with light sleep, whilst stage 3 is the deepest phase of sleep. During stage 3[37], tissue growth and repair occurs and hormones required for growth and development are released[38].

The first REM cycle occurs about 90 minutes after falling asleep and lasts for about ten minutes, dreams are most likely to occur during this phase of sleep[39].

The body is, if we listen to it, finely tuned to be sure you get enough sleep. Two factors let you know it is time to go to sleep:

- The level of the neurotransmitter adenosine in our blood

- Messages from our circadian clock

Adenosine is produced as a by-product of you expending energy during the day and is monitored by the brain. When adenosine levels rise we will feel drowsier, meanwhile decreased levels (as occurs when we're sleeping) increase alertness when we wake up. We can override this system with caffeine and other stimulants that effectively block the adenosine receptors in the brain, preventing the body from turning your 'dimmer switches' down. This will affect your ability to concentrate, recall and react to stimuli, and may disrupt your ability to fall asleep.

Our circadian clock regulates not only your sleep but also body temperature, blood pressure, and levels of certain key hormones. In general, most people have a sleepiness peak between 12 midnight and 6am, with a dip between 2pm and 4pm. But this varies with some of us being night owls and others up with the dawn.

Why do we need sleep?

According to a study by Oxford University and the Royal College for Public Health, four out of ten people in the UK aren't getting enough sleep. The consequences of this can be severe. The report reveals that only after a short period of reduced sleep, the body is more vulnerable to infection and reacts less well to vaccinations[40].

Lack of sleep, or erratic sleep patterns, also make it hard for the body to recuperate and impair cognitive function, affecting the memory, attention span and making it more likely that you will have an accident. Chronic sleep deprivation increases the risk of high blood pressure, coronary heart disease and stroke. People who don't get enough shut-eye are also more prone to obesity as lack of sleep affects the appetite-regulating hormones, leptin and ghrelin[41].

Another study by scientists at the University of Rochester revealed that sleep helps the brain to remove damaging toxins. In fact, while we're sleeping, the amount of fluid in the brain increases dramatically, allowing it to cleanse itself [42]. This might explain why we can't think straight when we're tired. How many people have made a bad decision based on lack of sleep?

Get a good night

In our frantic 24/7 lives, sleep can sometimes seem like a luxury. But a good night's rest is a necessity, and there are changes you can make to ensure you wake up feeling refreshed.

Evidence from various studies reveals that regular exercise helps adults to sleep better[43] although it may be best to stick to morning or afternoon workouts as exercising late in the evening can make it initially harder to nod off.

The best time to exercise, though, is whenever you want to exercise – we're all different, after all. Even the athletes among us are more likely to peak at different times of the day. This is determined by your internal body clock or circadian rhythms, according to research published in the journal *Current Biology*[44]. So, you need to check in with your body clock if you really want to feel rested. This means making the effort, within reason, to get up and go to bed at the same time each day.

Cutting back on gadgets, as we have seen before, will also help you to sleep better. A Harvard Medical School study has shown that the blue light from screens and devices inhibits the production of melatonin, the hormone that helps you sleep[45] (see Chapter 9).

If you're a coffee drinker, you may need to reduce your caffeine intake (that includes chocolate, fizzy drinks and tea too) at least six hours before bedtime[46] and limit yourself to two units of booze a day. As a stimulant, alcohol can keep you awake at night[47] (see Chapter 7 for a longer discussion on alcohol).

And if you have the chance to take a nap, do so. A study in 2014 by NASA revealed that a 40-minute nap improved alertness amongst its military pilots and astronauts by 100%[48].

Five steps to a better night's sleep:

- Ban devices from the bedroom

- Go to bed and get up at the same time

- Cut out coffee in the afternoon and go easy on alcohol

- Get plenty of exercise, preferably not within three hours of bedtime

- Schedule a nap into your day (especially useful for night owls and shift workers) if necessary, but not so long that it interferes with your ability to sleep at night

What is an ideal amount?

A long-standing sleep 'deficit' could well be charging long-term health 'interest' and whilst it may take some discipline to correct, it is possible. Only in the cases of extreme insomnia or other medical conditions will you need a doctor or drugs to help you.

The National Sleep Foundation says seven hours could be optimum for most adults[49]. Don't assume you can catch up on lost sleep, the best approach is to just get back into a routine. Anything over nine hours appears to be as bad as jet lag!

Free radicals

What exactly are free radicals? Without getting too bogged down in the chemistry, free radicals are molecules that carry an extra electron. This makes the compound more reactive as they rob electrons from healthy cells in your body to make up a pair, which can directly affect DNA and other molecules.

An excess of free radicals can damage DNA and causes your body to age. They also make us more vulnerable to heart disease and cancer[50].

Although free radicals are produced naturally in our bodies, it is believed that they can also come from the following sources:

- Pollution

- Alcohol

- High stress levels

- Pesticides

- UV rays

- Sugar

- Smoking

Antioxidants

Antioxidants are important as they can neutralise the extra electron reducing the level of free radicals and oxidative stress in your body thereby preventing cell damage. Be sure to include natural antioxidant-rich food in your diet, such as:

- Berries, cherries, plums, grapes, oranges and mangos

- Artichokes, cabbage, broccoli, asparagus, beetroot and spinach

- Pecan nuts, almonds, cashews and hazelnuts[50]

An antioxidant-rich diet can also reduce your health risk from air pollution, as the antioxidants protect you from nitrous oxide and other pollutants in the air [51].

So, this is simple: a diet full of fruit and vegetables will provide you with enough antioxidants. Or is it that simple? I am sure you have seen the proliferation of supplements and other products that claim to include antioxidants in their ingredients.

Antioxidants are a clear example of how science has been distorted by marketing departments to promote products. I want to explain this in full as a good example of how 'sciency' speak can be used to promote products.

The antioxidant craze started in 1981 when a study published in *Nature* showed a correlation between b-carotene and blood retinol (both antioxidants) inversely correlated with cancer rates. This made sense: free radicals react with DNA, causing mutations which give rise to cancer, so eliminating them with antioxidants would result in a lower cancer rate[52]. This idea captured the imaginations of marketing departments of cosmetics (anti-ageing and moisturising), cleaning and supplementation products. You will see the result of this marketing frenzy in the shops today.

However, two very large subsequent intervention studies showed the opposite: b-carotene, vitamin A and vitamin E groups had significantly higher lung cancer and overall death rates compared to the placebo[53]. Indeed, one study [54] had to be called off early as it was deemed too unethical to continue: the group taking antioxidant tablets had a 28% increase in lung cancer rate and 17% increase in death rate compared to the placebo group.

Two further Colchrane systematic unbiased metanalysis reviews of all the literature available showed that antioxidant supplements were ineffective[55], the most recent one even showing that supplements actually appear to increase mortality[56,57]. Despite this, marketing departments and some 'health' advocates have clung to their intuitions rather than examining scientific evidence, and still voraciously advocate antioxidants. Of course, these studies do not mean we should avoid foods with antioxidants, they are very beneficial when consumed via a healthy diet.

The scientific community has a high integrity, and this is reflected in the tradition of formally withdrawing research if subsequent studies show they are incorrect. The problem is once an idea hits the imaginations of marketing departments and is converted into amazing products, this integrity is lost and the connection between causation and correlation is ignored. The general public, will have no idea of the truth of the science unless they do what I have done and look at the research papers.

It is true that targeted antioxidant therapy has had some clinical use – for example, baicalein and catechins to treat osteoarthritis[58] – showing that antioxidants could still be beneficial to human health, and a clinical trial of Coenzyme Q10 seemed to support the fact that antioxidants can have a positive effect on vascular function.

Doug Seals, one of the researchers, said: "This study breathes new life into the discredited theory that supplementing diet with antioxidants can improve health." It showed that antioxidants can reverse the effect of ageing in our blood vessels, with participants performing as if they were 15/20 years younger and their artery dilation improved by 42%[59]. But this does not mean all antioxidant supplementation will do this, which is what the marketing people will have you believe!

As mentioned in Chapter 6, the consumption of known antioxidant-containing foods like turmeric has been distorted by media coverage, so it is important that all nutritional claims are backed up by correct scientific interpretation and, if there is insufficient evidence, that this is highlighted. The Alzheimer's Society says in a report that research supporting antioxidant supplements and the prevention of Alzheimer's is 'limited' and 'conflicting'[60] but do go on to advocate the consumption of fruit and vegetables. Getting your antioxidants through healthy fresh food will never be proved wrong.

I want to move on from this confusion created by the friction between science and intuition. Here are some everyday suggestions to increase your antioxidants without taking expensive supplements. Fruit and vegetables are high in antioxidants and have been shown to have countless health benefits, such as lowering your cancer risk [61]:

Juicing or blending?

My friend Regina asked why we should juice and not blend. My answer was to do both – would she ever eat ten carrots raw? Juicing will give you all the antioxidants in one glass!

I love juice, but juices should *never* be meal substitutes. They don't contain enough roughage. So why not buy a carton from the supermarket? Well, shop-bought juices aren't all as healthy as you might think, many are made from concentrate and have added sugar. For example, to make many of the shop-bought orange juices, they are first pasteurised (a process that destroys many of the nutrients) then heated, which makes the water evaporate. Producers may store this substance for months, and later mix water back in, adding other flavours and refined sugars to produce 'juice'. Definitely look for non-concentrated brands. If you make your own, the juicer squeezes out all the juice from the fruit or vegetables, so you get a high concentration of vitamins, minerals and antioxidants.

How to juice:

- Only juice organic fruits and vegetables; with non-organic fruit, make sure you peel them otherwise you may be concentrating the pesticides on the non-organic food into the juice; alternatively, stick to the 'Clean 15' fruit (see Chapter 2)

- Use a juicer that does not produce heat as this kills some of the nutrients

- Berries can make the juice a bit gloopy, so you might want to think twice before adding them to your juice

Contrary to what you might think, fruit and vegetables can definitely be juiced together. I love juicing ginger with a bag of carrots, celery, spinach, lemon, orange, and kale or any green vegetable you fancy. You can change the quantities to suit your individual taste.

Blending

A smoothie made in a blender is much thicker than a juice and can be used to replace a meal if necessary. A blender breaks down the entire fruit or vegetable to ensure that you get all the nutrients and fibre.

What can you add?

It is up to you. However, if you're looking for inspiration, here are a few common ingredients along with their respective benefits:

- Avocado (protein and fat)
- Ginger (anti-inflammatory)
- Lemon (antiseptic)
- Carrots (vitamin C)
- Flaxseed (zinc, iron and magnesium)
- Beetroot (vitamin C and potassium)
- Linseed or chia (omega-3 fatty acids)

Note: Ensure the chia seeds are fully hydrated or have been ground before you drink otherwise they will dehydrate you!

My favourite smoothie is made from half a courgette with a piece of ginger, a handful of kale, and half a pear or apple mixed with almond milk, coconut water or coconut milk. Add maca powder or bee pollen too. Enjoy! The RYG programme has delicious smoothies included for breakfast.

If this seems like too much hard work, try these simple detox drinks:

Lemon and cucumber: Just add chopped cucumber and lemon to a jug of water – simple. The antiseptic in the lemon mixed with the cucumber's antioxidant properties will help to detoxify the body.

Ginger detox tea: Make a cup of green tea with lemon, honey and ginger. This provides a cup full of goodness with the ginger aiding digestion.

To enema or not?

In this book I have used fully evidenced research, while occasionally referring to other, less investigated approaches. The enema is one of the 'other approaches'. I have a good friend who swears that having a regular enema in conjunction with juicing enabled him to head off obesity, failing energy and depression. I have been known to reach for my kit when I feel in need of an extra boost to clear out my system from modem life. Placebo or not, I have found that those who try it after initial reluctance turn into covert converts!

Presently orthodox medicine dismisses enemas, but this was not always the case. The oldest continuously published medical text book included the enema until 1972 when it was removed 'because of space consideration' [62]. Previously enemas have been used for post-operative care[63] and for shock after abdominal surgery.

How do they work? The theory is that an enema, like drinking coffee, stimulates the liver and gallbladder to increase the flow of bile, and this is supported by an experiment using a camera to look at the bile duct before and after the enema, showing the bile obstructing the camera's view had cleared.

The Gerson Therapy[64] that advocates the use of enemas and juice is based on the theory that cancer is caused by alteration of cell metabolism by toxic environmental substances and processed food due to changes in levels of sodium and potassium in the body. It emphasises increasing potassium intake and minimising sodium consumption to correct the electrolyte imbalance, repair tissue, and detoxify the liver. Coffee enemas are used to help the dilation of bile ducts and help the excretion of toxic breakdown products processed by the liver and through the colon wall[65]. It has been found by practitioners that coffee enemas have a sedative effect whilst stimulating the liver and gall bladder, and if you investigate the testimonials of cancer survivors they are inspiring.

I was recently asked to demonstrate how to do an enema at an 'Eat to Beat Cancer Workshop' (fully clothed!) by the nutritionist and type 4 breast cancer survivor Jenny Philips. You can buy the kit from www. gerson.org.Please follow the instructions carefully if you decide to do it at home, but it is incredibly simple.

An enema is very different from colonic irrigation – typically offered at health clinics – which claims to detoxify the body, normalise intestinal function, treat IBS and help weight loss. None of these claims seemed to be supported by sound scientific evidence and the claims may well be misleading[66].

Summing up

- Drink between six and eight glasses of water a day
- Ensure that your diet provides you with all essential nutrients and fibre
- Eat natural Viagra
- Try fasting
- Have regular sleeping hours

Fight free radicals by stacking your diet with fresh food full of antioxidants (not supplements).

Notes:

CHAPTER 14

Create your own Blue Zone!

You may already be putting into action the suggestions made in this book, and this will do you no harm, or you will be ready to start right now!

Can I encourage you by telling you about the five areas in the world called Blue Zones that provide a great model of how to live a longer and happier life?

If you haven't heard of Blue Zones before, these are areas in the world that have been identified as the healthiest places to live. People from these areas typically remain active well into their eighties[1], generally remain healthier for longer without the need for medication, and are ten times more likely to reach 100 than those living in most parts of the USA.

So far, five Blue Zones have been identified: the Italian island of Sardinia, Okinawa in Japan, Loma Linda in California, the Greek island of Ikaria and Costa Rica's Nicoya Peninsula[1].

So, what's their secret?

Overwhelmingly, they have taken responsibility for what they eat and do not eat a standard western diet. They are outside of any typical medical environment because they eat to live not live to eat.

Dr Sarah McKay states that for those who survive over 100, "30% is to do with genetics and 70% is to do with lifestyle". [1]

There are certain lifestyle factors that these long-living communities have in common[1,2]:

- A healthy diet with an emphasis on plant-based foods

- An active lifestyle, moving naturally

- Managing stress

- A strong sense of connection, purpose and 'resilience and optimism'

- The 80:20 rule: 80% great lifestyle with a leeway of 20% for when we stray!

A healthy diet

Our body is designed to be supported by good nutritious food. This is the energy it needs to communicate within itself and function effectively.

The Blue Zone diets are largely made up of vegetables, fruit, fish, nuts and pulses, people rarely eat meat and dairy products and hardly ever have processed food. This is the same as the Mediterranean diet and the RYG programme is based on this approach.

It's not surprising then that the people who live in these areas are so healthy, especially as they get older.

The World Health Organisation estimates that a staggering 80% of premature deaths from heart disease and stroke could be preventable with simple lifestyle changes[3]. Furthermore, there is extensive evidence to suggest that risks of other diseases, such as diabetes, Alzheimer's and cancer can be reduced with a healthy diet [4-7].

Re-read Chapter 2 for advice about eating well.

An active lifestyle

Although older people living in the Blue Zones may not have gym memberships, research shows that they naturally build exercise into their everyday lives, and rarely sit down. In Japan's Okinawa, even older people spend a lot of time each day in their gardens, tending to their home-grown fruit and vegetables. They are also keen walkers, and they eat all their meals sitting on the floor – all that getting up and down every day increases their upper body strength, making them less vulnerable to falling down[2].

The NHS recommends that to help prevent illness, healthy people over the age of 65 should either do 75 minutes of vigorous aerobic exercise a week, such as playing tennis or running, or 150 minutes of moderate aerobic exercise like cycling or walking. They should also include strength exercises that work all the major muscles two or three days a week[8].

In our non-Blue Zone lives, inactivity seems to have reached shocking levels: one 2013 study revealed that almost 80% of the population fails to hit exercise target guidelines[2]. In Chapter 3 we looked at the benefits of exercise in detail.

Managing stress

Research has revealed that people living in the Blue Zones don't necessarily have less stressful lives, but they are better equipped to deal with life's ups and downs. Not only are these communities more connected and family orientated, they also have healthy practices for relieving stress. The Californian Seventh Day Adventists pray; the Ikarians take regular naps; the Sardinians have almost daily family get-togethers. If these are not practical, create your own healthy stress-beating strategies to make your life feel as calm and rounded as possible.

Around 12 million people in the UK visit their GP with stress every year, and according to the latest research from the Office of National Statistics, one in four adults suffer from either anxiety or depression. Concerns over debt, job security, fragile relationships, bereavement and the trend for aspirational living are some of the many issues that appear to be driving the stress epidemic.

Stress, as we have seen, has a physical effect on our body, causing the release of hormones (adrenaline and cortisol). Although stress has an important and natural role in our lives, when we are under constant stress it can be very detrimental to our health, causing digestive issues, headaches, high blood pressure, inflammation, reduced immune function and an increased risk of heart attack and stroke[3,4,5].

I hope you are now a bit more aware of the challenges of 21st century living and understand the importance of:

- Changing some of your lifestyle choices

- Balancing your gut bacteria before other interventions

- The influence your physical health has on your mental health

- That your health will not get better by chance, it gets better by change

Good luck, listen to your body, you only have one, and keep me posted on any successes and challenges.

Go and create your own Blue Zone!

About the author

Catherine Rogers is the founder of www.maphealthsolutions.com, an innovative practice that focuses on the way physical health can improve mental health. An integrative therapist, she uses CBT, EFT and NLP in conjunction with improving physical wellbeing. She is passionate about this approach and aims to be a thought leader in this embryonic field, especially emphasising how important the health of gut bacteria is to our mental and physical health.

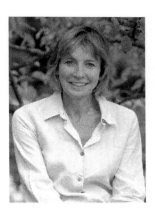

In a varied career, Catherine has worked in many different environments ranging from the City of London and Oxford University to the jungles of Guyana. She has written a book about her time in the jungle called *Reckless* which will be published in 2020. She is now applying her honed problem-solving abilities to the rising tide of chronic health conditions. She has realised that it isn't that people don't understand what constitutes a healthy lifestyle, the problem is that they don't know how to do it.

To show how, she has created an informative and affordable online course called *Reset Your Gut* to accompany this book, so as well as understanding the theory, readers will have a practical course showing how to get their gut back on track. It has been written with the help of nutritionists, dieticians, doctors, recipe writers and scientists and includes recipe plans for any food preferences and guidelines as to how to incorporate it into your life going forward, see www.ryghealth.com.

Her favourite saying is: "A problem is only a problem because it has a solution, and if you are not thinking of the solution, you are part of the problem."

Catherine lives in Oxfordshire with Chris, her 'rock' of a husband. They have three children, Jack, Annie and Mia, who are the driving force in her life.

Printed in Great
Britain
by Amazon